W9-CFB-073

Chicken Soup for the Soul
Healthy Living:
Weight Loss

Jack Canfield

Mark Victor Hansen

Andrew Larson, M.D.
AUTHOR, *THE GOLD COAST CURE*

Health Communications, Inc.
Deerfield Beach, Florida

www.hcibooks.com
www.chickensoup.com

We would like to acknowledge the many publishers and individuals who granted us permission to reprint the cited material.

I Learned It from My Dog reprinted by permission of Kirsten Mortensen. ©2004 Kirsten Mortensen.

Don't Give Up, Don't Ever Give Up reprinted by permission of Amy Westlake, N.D. ©2004 Amy Westlake, N.D.

Start Living Now reprinted by permission of Vicki Jeffries. ©2004 Vicki Jeffries.

Diets Don't Work But This Does reprinted by permission of Mary Silver. ©2004 Mary Silver.

(Continued on page 132)

Library of Congress Cataloging-in-Publication Data
available from the Library of Congress

©2005 Jack Canfield and Mark Victor Hansen
ISBN 0-7573-0277-7

Publisher: Health Communications, Inc.
          3201 S.W. 15th Street
          Deerfield Beach, FL 33442-8190

Cover design by Larissa Hise Henoch
Inside book design by Lawna Patterson Oldfield
Inside book formatting by Dawn Von Strolley Grove

Contents

Fear less, hope more,

eat less, chew more,

whine less, breathe more,

talk less, say more,

love more,

and all good things

will be yours.

—Swedish Proverb

Introduction:
Your Weight Is Within Your Control

There are many reasons to lose weight. Maybe your doctor has told you that you need to lose weight to improve your health. Maybe you just found out your cholesterol level is too high and you need to improve your eating and exercising routine to protect your heart. Perhaps you are tired of looking at those "thin" jeans you used to fit into and you want to actually wear them again. Maybe you find yourself no longer able to keep up with your little ones like you used to. No matter what your reason for wanting to lose weight, you'll find useful, inspirational advice in this book.

Losing weight is not simply a matter of looking thinner. Excess weight is the driving force behind a recent explosion in the incidence of Type II diabetes. Excess weight increases your risk of having a heart attack, developing cancer and spending time in the hospital. Just as important, carrying excess weight makes it harder to enjoy the little things in life like golfing, shopping, traveling and playing with your children and grandchildren.

I know it's not easy but I'm here to convince you

that your weight is within your control. It is possible to make tremendous strides toward improving your health and your image if you're willing to make the effort. This book is filled with inspirational success stories and invaluable medical, nutritional and lifestyle advice designed to maximize your chance for achieving success.

No matter how frustrated you might be, no matter how fed up you are, now is not the time to give up. If the number of people who are overweight can increase, the number can decrease, too. *You* can be one of the many people who succeed at losing weight. The logic really is that simple.

Why do people gain weight? Many factors have been blamed, but only a few of these explanations make sense. For instance, people sometimes blame their genes. But the fact is genes don't change much over the years. If genetics were to blame there wouldn't be an epidemic. The same number of people would be overweight now as were overweight in any other era of prosperity.

Stress, psychology and hormones have been blamed. But doctors are very good at manipulating hormones. Just look at the strides we've made in treating breast cancer, thyroid disease and infertility. If hormones were primarily responsible for weight gain we'd be winning that war too.

Does stress cause weight gain? Probably not. As stressful as our lives may seem today, think about how stressful it must have been to live in a world without cars, without running water and without being able to call 911. It's almost impossible to argue that the stresses of contemporary living are primarily to blame for today's obesity epidemic.

The good news is that factors you *can* change are primarily to blame for those extra pounds. You can choose to eat more healthful foods. You can choose to exercise. You can choose to associate with people who are supportive of your efforts to lose weight. You can learn about positive lifestyle change without spending hundreds of dollars on special programs, without reading boring textbooks, without scouring the far reaches of the World Wide Web. *Chicken Soup for the Soul Healthy Living* is all about turning the tables. *Chicken Soup* challenges and inspires you to take control of your life, your health and your spirit.

As a physician who devotes a significant part of his practice to treating the medical and surgical consequences of obesity, I stand 100 percent behind the advice in this book, and the messages of hope in these pages. It is possible to learn from every single person who has taken the time to contribute his or her story.

I wish you well as you achieve success. Here's to healthy living!

Andrew Larson, M.D.
Author, *The Gold Coast Cure*

I Learned It from My Dog

A nswers can come from unexpected places: I learned how to overcome my weight problem from my dog.

It was nearly thirty years ago. Brett was an Irish setter–Doberman mix, and she was bright, high-spirited and willful—the sort of temperament that, unfortunately, made her a poor choice in pets for a teenager whose understanding of dog training was based primarily on the Irish Red books. Brett was nearly impossible to control. Whether it was climbing on forbidden furniture, refusing to come when called or barking her head off when a doorbell rang, no lesson I tried to teach her seemed to catch on. My attempts at discipline were met with constant failure. I loved the dog. She was my best friend. But her wildness infuriated and exhausted me.

Then one night, I had a dream. . . . But I'll come back to that in a minute.

First, my weight.

I'd been thin as a kid. But somewhere between age sixteen and nineteen, I started to put on the extra pounds. In retrospect, I know I fell into an all-too-common trap.

It started when I became convinced I had an ugly body. The biggest problem was my chest. It was way too small. Night after night I'd study my profile in a full-length mirror, hoping my shape would suddenly appear more shapely. No such luck. I stopped growing somewhere shy of a full B cup and that was that.

It seemed like such an awful fate. Surely, if I were only bigger, my life would be heaven. The boys I liked would like me back. I'd be invited to the really cool parties. I'd be the envy of the most popular kids in the school.

Mirrors are delusive things. Stare at yourself too long and features that are perfectly normal shift and swell. They appear suddenly disproportionate and exaggerated. That's exactly what my mirror-staring did to me: it began to look as if part of the problem was that my stomach stuck out too much. Suck my stomach in, I noticed, and my bust looked bigger.

A flatter stomach, that's what I needed! The trap was sprung. I decided to diet.

My diet was typical for the 1970s. I counted calories. But I found myself woefully devoid of willpower. One day I'd do great, keeping my intake to 1,000 calories or less. But the next day, off the deep end I'd go. I'd binge like a starving person. Boxes of cookies, huge dishes of ice cream (my favorite trick was to pour mounds of bittersweet chocolate chips over three or four scoops of vanilla ice cream), bags of Doritos. I'd often eat so much rich food that I'd feel nauseous afterward—yet I seemed powerless to stop myself. No matter how much I hated the part of me that gorged on those forbidden treats, no matter how much I scolded myself, no matter what promises I made, I couldn't stop. It was like I was two people. And when the one that wanted to binge took over, the dieter was shoved off in a corner where she couldn't utter a peep. My frustration was agonizing. I began to suspect I wanted to be fat. That same perverse psychological phenomenon was running—and ruining—my life.

My worst fears began to come true. In a few short years, I went from about 115 pounds to over 145. None of which, by the way, settled on my bust!

It was then that I had the dream about my dog.

In the dream Brett—who in real life had a beautiful red-brown coat—was not brown at all. Instead, she kept changing back and forth from white to black and back to white. And her color, in the dream, depended entirely on me. When I scolded her, calling her a bad dog, she turned black. When I called her a good dog and praised her, she became white.

The next morning I thought about the dream,

and quickly realized what it was trying to tell me. My style of discipline wasn't working, because instead of preventing my dog's "bad" behavior, I was reinforcing it. I expected a bad dog, treated her as if she were a bad dog, and so—she was a bad dog.

I immediately began handling Brett differently. I started ignoring her when she did something I didn't like. Then, when she did the "right" thing— when she came when I called, for example— I praised her with complete love and enthusiasm.

The transformation was stunning. Suddenly, my dog was "obeying" me. Oh, she was still often a handful—excitable, restless and a bit too intelligent to ever really settle down completely—but we found ourselves getting along much better. It turns out, you see, that most of the time she really wanted to please me. I just needed to nurture her good behavior. The rest took care of itself.

Then, one day, I realized I'd been treating *myself* as poorly as I had once treated my pet. I was beating myself up every time I ate something "fattening." I was calling myself undisciplined, fat, a failure. I was reinforcing, on a daily basis, the exact image I most feared and disliked. Suddenly, I understood why I binged—I was simply being the person I constantly told myself I was. Weak. An overeater. Out of control.

From that day, I never punished myself again

about a single morsel of food. Instead, I began noticing how often I ate good, nutritious meals. I began getting excited about how eating right made me feel great. I began taking pleasure in learning about whole foods. I indulged in my interest in cooking and began to collect recipes and cookbooks.

When I did eat something "fattening," I enjoyed it as I ate, then put it quickly out of my mind. If I caught myself later regretting that slice of cake or ice-cream bar, I told myself firmly to just let it go.

And guess what happened? Food and eating gradually lost that intense emotional charge they'd once had. When I ate, more and more it was because I was hungry and something appealed to me. I began to trust my body's signals. I quit counting calories, I quit weighing myself (to this day, I don't keep a scale in the house; I know I'm "thin" but I couldn't tell you how much I weigh).

I didn't lose the extra pounds overnight. In fact, it took several years. But by my mid-twenties, the new self I'd created—the one that eats for the right reasons, in the right quantities—had become my "real" self.

There are many variations among people's physiologies and body chemistries. There may not be any "one size fits all" diet everyone can use to reach their ideal weight. But my experience taught me one thing for certain: anybody can create a weight problem, or make a weight problem worse, if the only feedback they give themselves is negative.

Instead, we have to treat ourselves with love and compassion. We have to nourish the good, not waste all our energy trying to stamp out the bad.

So, here's to the memory of my old friend, Brett. What a lifelong gift she turned out to be!

♥ *Kirsten Mortensen*

You Can Do It!

You may have tried to lose weight many times before. If you've tried dieting, you may even have lost weight, only to gain it right back again. Whether this is your first time or your tenth time trying to lose weight, here's the good news: You CAN lose weight permanently. You don't have to starve yourself or exercise for hours on end every day. By making just a few healthy, lasting changes in the way you live your life, you can start looking and feeling better right away. You can lose weight and keep the pounds off for a lifetime.

Improve Your Health

There are plenty of reasons to lose weight, but the most important is to improve your health. If you are even slightly overweight, you're more likely to develop all sorts of serious health problems such as:

- heart disease
- stroke
- diabetes
- cancer (such as colon cancer, endometrial cancer, and postmenopausal breast cancer)
- gallbladder disease
- sleep apnea (interrupted breathing during sleep)
- osteoarthritis (wearing away of the joints)

Take it from a doctor with years of clinical experience. Obesity makes almost any disease more difficult to treat. Operations take longer and anesthesia is much more risky when you are overweight.

The good news is even a very modest amount of weight loss—10 to 15 pounds—offers significant health benefits. Some people with Type II diabetes are cured by losing only a small amount of weight. It doesn't take much to make a big difference so far as your health is concerned. Lose weight for your health first!

Lowering Your Cholesterol Level and Blood Pressure

Don't let appearances deceive you. You don't even have to be overweight to suffer from many of the medical conditions that can be improved by the lifestyle advice in this book. For example, you can be thin and still have a high cholesterol level or high blood pressure. In this case, in order to protect your heart, you'll most definitely want to follow the advice in this book about eating healthfully and exercising properly. Some people are able to lower their cholesterol level and blood pressure sufficiently through lifestyle changes alone. Talk with your doctor about it—medicine is not always necessary.

It Can Be Done!

The National Weight Control Registry is a research study that has proven it is possible to achieve significant, long-term weight loss. The registry has identified more than 4,000 people who have lost at least 30 pounds and have maintained a weight loss of at least 30 pounds for one year or longer. The registry researchers report that:

- ❤ Nearly every participant used diet and exercise to initially lose weight and maintain their weight loss.
- ❤ Weight loss led to significant improvements in self-confidence, mood, and physical health.
- ❤ About half of registry members initially lost weight on their own; the rest used a formal weight-loss program or help from a health-care professional.

- ♥ Once you've successfully maintained your new weight for several years, the chances increase that you'll maintain that weight.
- ♥ Eating breakfast is a characteristic common to successful weight loss and may be a factor in success.
- ♥ People who stick to their new eating plan throughout the week are 150 percent more likely to maintain their weight over the subsequent year than people who diet mostly on weekdays.

⌛ *Think about* . . .
why I want to lose weight

The reasons I want to lose weight are:

❏ To feel better

❏ To have more energy

❏ To lower my cholesterol

❏ To reduce my risk of diabetes

❏ To reduce my risk of a heart attack

❏ To look better

❏ To live longer

❏ _____

❏ _____

❏ _____

Don't Give Up, Don't Ever Give Up

"Lucille, after reviewing your lab results, you have a condition known as fatty liver. What this means is that your liver is turning to fat. I have good news and bad news. We'll start with the bad news. If you do not do anything about this, your liver will continue to turn to fat, you will develop cirrhosis of the liver, and you will die of liver failure. The good news is that this condition is completely reversible. The liver is a very resilient organ, and it has a great ability to heal itself. There is only one way to reverse this condition. You must lose 30 pounds."

I could see the look of terror on Lucille's face. I have found one of the hardest parts of being a doctor is to tell someone they must lose weight, not for their outer appearance or self-esteem, but for their health. There is no magic pill to take away the symptoms or the reality of this condition. Losing weight is a matter of will from within. As a doctor, you cannot just write a prescription and send the patient out the door and off to the pharmacy. You must become their life coach.

"Doctor, I've tried to lose weight for over three years. I've tried every plan out there. I lose a little, and then I gain it all back. There must be something else I can do," Lucille explained with a slight hint of panic in her voice.

I rolled my chair over to Lucille's chair, with our knees almost touching, and looked deeply into her eyes. "Have you really wanted to lose weight?" Lucille broke our gaze as she turned her attention down towards the floor. There was silence. She slowly began to lift her head and I noticed a tear forming in her left eye.

"I . . . I have never had a reason to lose weight. I am unattractive; my husband and I divorced over ten years ago; no one pays any attention to me. . . ."

Lucille's tears began to flow. "Doctor, are you telling me I am going to die?" I grabbed Lucille's hand. "No, Lucille. You are going to lose weight." Lucille looked up from the floor. She looked at me as if I was the only person in years to have faith in her. I even noticed a slight smile forming on her lips. "How do I do it? Do you have a special diet plan?"

"It is not another diet that you need. You have tried them already. They worked for a while, but they were unsustainable. Our job is to discover why they were unsustainable and then develop strategies to overcome the pitfalls. We are going to develop lifelong habits, not only eating and exercise habits, but habits that make you feel whole and healthy as a person. This isn't going to be easy, but it's going to be worth it.

"But before we begin we must both, you and I, agree to a motto on this new life journey of yours. The motto has been a favorite of mine since spoken by former North Carolina State coach Jimmy Valvano as he was dying of cancer. 'Don't give up, don't ever give up.'"

Lucille and I saw each other every month for the next two years. I even received phone calls from her at odd hours of the day and night. By the end of two years, Lucille had gone from 205 pounds to 170. She had exceeded our goal of 30 pounds and she wasn't slowing down. She was determined that she was going to reach a weight that made her feel healthy and whole.

At our two-year visit as Lucille stood on the scale, she reached over and grabbed my left hand with her right. "Thank you for believing in me so I could believe in myself. You are making a difference."

As she walked out the door that day, she turned, looked over her shoulder and recaptured the gaze we had shared many times over the past two years. "Don't give up," she said. "Don't ever give up." I don't know if she was talking to herself or to me.

♥ *Amy Westlake, N.D.*

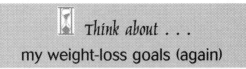

Think about . . .
my weight-loss goals (again)

What is my ideal weight?

What is my weight-loss goal per week?

How long do I think it will take me to get down to my ideal weight?

What do I plan to do to get there?

Am I willing to eat more fruits and vegetables?

Am I willing to exercise more every week?

Am I willing to talk about my weight-loss goals with friends and loved ones?

My Page

My Thoughts _____

_____

_____

_____

My Feelings _____

_____

_____

_____

My Facts _____

_____

_____

_____

My Support _____

_____

_____

Weight-Loss Goals

Setting the right goals can make all the difference in your success or failure, so always:

- **Set goals for changing your lifestyle,** rather than losing a specific number of pounds. If you eat healthfully and exercise, you will improve your life in a number of ways, not just by losing pounds.
- **Make your lifestyle goals specific.** It's easy to say, "I'll eat more fruits and vegetables," but you're more likely to stick to the plan when your goal is, "I'll have a fruit salad with my lunch every day this week."
- **Make your goals measurable.** Instead of saying, "I want to be more fit," say, "I want to be able to walk for an hour without getting winded."
- **Choose a realistic way of reaching your goal.** If you eventually want to exercise for an hour a day, start with a goal of twenty minutes three times a week, and work up to an hour slowly.
- **Don't make your goals too rigid.** Who could possibly stick to a goal of "I'll never eat sweets again"? Instead, say, "I'll start by substituting a piece of fruit for that vending-machine candy bar I've gotten into the habit of eating at work."

- **Set a time limit for achieving your goals,** or you may never get around to them.
- **Pick a reward for meeting your goals,** such as, "If I meet my exercise goal for this week, I'll treat myself to a movie on Saturday night."

Some of you have a goal in mind. Before reading further, let's make sure your goal is medically appropriate and realistic. One way of getting a handle on what your weight should be is to use the doctor's preferred tool, the *Body Mass Index* (BMI) chart for adults. Measure your weight and height, then see where you fall on the chart following.

The Winning Attitude

Be realistic, and be flexible, with your goal weight. You may get close to, but not quite hit, your target, yet still find you've lost enough weight to feel better, look better and be healthier. Many people find it easier to aim for several smaller goals about their meals, snacks, exercise habits, eating out and other areas. If you try this approach, you won't feel all is lost when you temporarily slip up in one area.

Ideal Body Weight—Weight in Pounds

Height in Feet and Inches	120	130	140	150	160	170	180	190	200	210	220	230	240	250
4'6"														
4'8"														
4'10"														
5'0"														
5'2"														
5'4"														
5'6"														
5'8"														
5'10"														
6'0"														
6'2"														
6'4"														
6'6"														
6'8"														

Overweight

Healthy Weight

Think about . . .
my weight-loss goals

My goal weight was:

My healthy weight is between:

The amount of weight I need to lose to get into the Healthy Weight category is:

Now that I've seen the Ideal Body Weight chart, my goal weight is:

Here's a small goal I know I can achieve in my first week of weight loss: _____

_____

Here's a medium-sized goal I'm pretty sure I can achieve in my first month: _____

_____

Here's a dream goal I'd love to achieve in six months:

_____

_____

My Page

My Thoughts _____

_____

_____

_____

My Feelings _____

_____

_____

_____

My Facts _____

_____

_____

_____

My Support _____

_____

_____

_____

Start Living Now

Twelve years ago I was in my last year of college, working, and as heavy as ever. I don't know how many pounds over the 200 mark I was because I didn't have the nerve to get on the scale, but I do know that I routinely got through studying for my finals with the help of a large fast-food value meal and a soda.

It had always been that food was my only consolation. I grew up a victim of child sexual abuse and domestic violence and became overweight at a young age. I dreaded going to school because of what the other kids would say. "Look, a fat chink!" one third-grade boy would always say to his friend, laughing loudly. It just didn't go together, being Asian and fat. My parents weren't much help, either. My mom piled the food on my plate at the same time she told me I ate too much. My dad just pitied me. I began to see myself as grotesquely ugly, and I spent my adolescence practicing the art of self-loathing. I fantasized about the day I would surprise everyone with my thin, beautiful body. The boys would be in love with me, the girls would be jealous, and everyone who had ever snickered at me would be so sorry for having done so.

Irene worked in the office next to me for almost two years. We were never the closest of friends, but we shared a lot of conversations over the years. She was in her early thirties, had never had a boyfriend, and still lived with her parents. She was overweight and frumpy looking. The other people we worked with laughed behind her back about how much she ate. Sure, she brought diet meals for dinner, but she always ate two of them at a time! "What good does that do?" they would laughingly question each other.

I knew Irene was a terrific person. Having come from a close family myself, I admired how she talked so lovingly about her parents and sister. She seemed to live vicariously through her sister, always recounting tales of her brother-in-law and niece and their happy suburban life. She never seemed to have any tales from her own life, though, and I knew what that was like. I had a pretty sister too. In fact, I felt like I could relate to Irene in a lot of ways. We both had weight issues. We both longed to step out onto the stage as stars in our own right.

A couple of months after I graduated from school and moved back home, a mutual friend of ours called me on the telephone. She told me Irene had been driving to work when a semitruck had pulled out in front of her. Her car slammed into the semi and she was killed instantly. The passenger in the truck's cab rushed to her side to help her, but she was already gone. The police dispatcher taking the call of the fatal accident had known Irene from work. She cried as she called to tell my ex-boss that Irene had been killed. I was devastated.

Immediately after Irene's death, I committed myself to getting serious about living my life actively rather than sitting on the sidelines. I had already wasted too much time being unhappy with myself and doing nothing to change my self-image. I started going to a health club every other day; I walked on the treadmill, lifted weights, swam, and relaxed in the hot tub and sauna. On my off days, I rode a stationary bike. It became routine for me. And it was more than just physically therapeutic; I talked to my mind and listened to my heart as I exercised. I made the changes for myself, but also for Irene. Irene showed me that I couldn't take for granted that the opportunity to start living the way I had dreamed would always be in front of me. She lost her opportunity, so I wanted to share my success with her. I lost ninety pounds over the next year and attained the best health of my life.

Now, twelve years later, I have a happy home with four beautiful children and a husband who is in love with me. I have just completed my master's degree. I have maintained my good health by walking forty minutes a day, five times a week. I feel strong and in charge of my life. I think that Irene has been here with me all the while, showing me that the time to start living is now.

❤ *Vicki Jeffries*

A New Attitude

You know you have to eat less and exercise more in order to lose weight, right? But if it was really that simple, everyone would be thin. We know it's not easy. But YOU CAN DO IT. Every day, people make the decision to lose weight, maybe for the first time, maybe for the fiftieth time. One of those times, it's going to stick. Make it this time!

Sure, it won't be easy. You find yourself in situations where tempting foods call out your name. Your busy lifestyle seems too packed to fit in exercise. But once you decide to take control of your life, you can make it happen.

In order for your weight-loss dream to become a reality, you need to:

- **Make a lifelong commitment.** If you simply plan to change your eating and exercise habits long enough to lose twenty pounds, then go back to your old ways, beware. Those twenty pounds will creep right back. You need to commit yourself to lifelong change.

- **Consider the timing.** Are you tackling other weighty matters—marriage or financial problems, for instance? If so, this may not be the best time to also try to lose weight. You need all your available mental and physical energy to make lifelong changes and stick with them. Try to find one or two quiet months so you can really put forth your best effort to work healthy living into your routine.

- **Know in advance you will on occasion slip up.** Nobody's perfect. Decide in advance how you're going to deal with the inevitable slip. The most important thing is not to let a relapse become an excuse for giving up.
- **Decide to lose weight for yourself.** If you're trying to lose weight to satisfy someone else, instead of to make yourself happy, you're much less likely to make your change a permanent one.
- **Keep your eye on your goals**. To lose weight, have more energy and improve your health, don't lose sight of your goals.

Too Good to Be True?

Don't let anyone convince you that you can lose weight without any effort. It's best to avoid:

- **Very low calorie diets.** They deprive you of important nutrients, burn muscle and slow your metabolism. These diets should be followed only in rare situations under medical supervision.
- **Very low carbohydrate diets.** These diets may

work in the short term but they hardly ever
result in permanent weight loss. You lose
weight quickly, only to regain it once you start
eating normally again. There are serious health
risks associated with "elimination" diets.

- **Fad diets.** Pineapples? Diet shakes? Food combining? Forget it.
- **Over-the-counter weight-loss products** such as diet patches, "fat blockers" or "starch blockers." If they worked, doctors would prescribe them!

Think about . . .
making eating changes

Those first steps you must take to make permanent changes in your eating habits may seem difficult, but there are so many things you can do to make things easier. Start with two items from the following list and keep working until you've checked them all off:

❏ I will get junk foods out of my house so they won't keep tempting me.

❏ I will have plenty of healthy snacks around such as fruits and vegetables (fresh, frozen, or canned), nuts and low-fat cheese.

❏ I will meet new people through a healthy-cooking class, or cook a healthy meal and invite friends over.

❏ I will buy a new food magazine, or ask a friend for a new recipe.

❏ I will make my weight-loss plan a good excuse to try out novel restaurants such as the new ethnic restaurant in town advertising its healthy, spicy fare.

❏ I pledge to eat breakfast every day so I won't be hungry later in the day.

My Page

My Thoughts _____

_____

_____

_____

My Feelings _____

_____

_____

_____

My Facts _____

_____

_____

_____

My Support _____

_____

_____

_____

Should I Get Professional Help?

There are many resources in your community to help you lose weight. An obvious place to start is your family doctor. If you would prefer receiving help from a doctor who deals primarily in weight loss, ask around to locate a specialist in bariatric medicine. The American Society of Bariatric Physicians lists hundreds of member physicians on their Web site (*www.asbp.org*). Particularly experienced weight-loss physicians often choose to become certified by the American Board of Bariatric Medicine, a credential of distinction in the field.

Many local hospitals have wellness clinics on campus with nutritionists and nurses on staff who are specially trained to help patients lose weight. Your employer or your health insurance provider may be able to enroll you in one of these programs at a substantial discount, especially if you can get your doctor to prescribe weight-loss therapy.

Diets Don't Work But This Does

It's a very odd thing—
As odd as can be—
That whatever Miss T. eats
Turns into Miss T.

WALTER DE LA MARE

Diets don't work. I know because I dieted for years and ended up fatter than before I started. Fatter and more depressed.

When I first decided to stop dieting, I was terrified I would blow up and look like the Goodyear blimp. I had dieted for so many years that I no longer trusted myself around food. It was scary but I told myself I would try not dieting for one week. Just one week.

Before I stopped dieting, I did one other thing. I changed my language and my mind-set. I told myself I was simply going to eat sensibly and well. No foods were forbidden. In fact, the only thing forbidden was the word *diet*.

That first small change meant I skipped my usual

say-goodbye-to-all-the-fattening-foods ritual. So I didn't begin my eating plan five pounds heavier because of my good-bye binge of chips, cookies, and other goodies before I started my diet.

Second, instead of focusing on food, I focused on my eating habits. I repeatedly told myself I was overweight not because I was a bad person, but because I had bad eating habits. And habits can be changed—slowly and patiently.

I chose one small thing to change. I had read that people who skip breakfast tend to eat more later in the day when the body is less able to process calories. I made sure to begin each day with a bowl of oatmeal with milk and blueberries that filled me up, not out. That made it easier to pass on the doughnuts or cupcakes that many of my coworkers had with their coffee.

Although I had originally come from clean-your-plate country, I decided it was time to emigrate. No matter what my mother told me when I was growing up, finishing everything on my plate would not help the starving children elsewhere in the world. I made it a rule to leave at least one bite of food on the plate. That forced me to pay attention to what I was eating, rather than eat mindlessly. I often found that I could leave two, three or even more bites if I listened to my stomach, rather than the TV, while I ate.

I experimented with other behaviors that made eating sensibly easier for me. I only ate while sitting down at the table, which allowed me to eat mindfully rather than unconsciously. Instead of using a dinner plate, I used a salad plate. Smaller portions didn't look as small, and by fooling my eyes I fooled my stomach, too.

I used the same idea with my favorite treats. I bought single-sized portions of chips and other foods that I craved. I found that just a small amount of the food was often enough to take away the craving. In some cases, where I couldn't get a single size, I limited those treats to restaurants rather than keeping them in the house where I might be tempted to overeat.

I worked in small increments and set realistic goals. I chose one new behavior to work on at a time. Instead of telling myself I would do this new behavior every day without fail, I aimed for two or three times a week. That way if I missed a day, it wasn't the end of the world. When I was confident I could do it two or three times a week, I increased the number of times until the new behavior became a habit.

I waited three or four weeks before working on a new habit because it takes that long for a new behavior to become ingrained. Introducing new patterns too soon wouldn't give me enough time to work on the ones I was already doing.

And the last thing I did was change the way I treated myself. I learned to be kind to myself, to give myself a break if I backslid or to hold off working on a new change if the timing simply wasn't right.

This technique was slow and I didn't lose all the weight in a day, a week or even a month. But I hadn't put it on that way either. It had crept up over the years and now it was going to come off the same way: slow and steady. But by looking at weight loss as a lifestyle change, by focusing on my behavior, and by making small, sustainable changes, the weight has continued to come off.

I'm within five pounds of my goal weight. Now that's what I call a success story.

♥ *Mary Silver*

Create a New Way to Eat

Your Friend: Whole Foods

With so many popular diets available it's easy to get caught up in the low-carb versus low-fat debate. Don't. Instead, concentrate on the quality of the foods you eat. If you eat "whole" foods high in protein, fiber and natural fats instead of processed foods you'll lose weight. Fiber, especially, fills you up and slows down the absorption of sugar into your bloodstream. This helps stabilize your blood sugar level and reduce cravings. High-fiber foods such as fruits, vegetables, beans and whole-grain products tend to be low in calories as well. When you eat healthy "whole" foods rich in the nutrients your body needs, you naturally regulate your appetite, lose weight and protect your body against disease.

Examples of whole foods include:

- chicken
- milk
- meat
- olives
- eggs
- yogurt with no sugar added
- strawberries
- whole-grain bread
- just about any food that isn't packaged

The Enemy: Processed Foods

When it comes to losing weight, processed foods, especially processed foods made with white flour and sugar, are the main roadblock. First, these foods don't have enough of the filling nutrients and fiber your body needs. Second, they can cause your blood sugar level to spike too high, then drop too low. Whenever your blood sugar level is low you get hungry and you eat more even though your body might not need those extra calories.

Culprit #1: Refined (Enriched) Flour

Refined flours are made from grains but they contain very little—less than 20 percent—of the nutrients, and none of the filling fiber, found in the natural whole grains from which they are made. Most packaged food products are made primarily from refined or enriched flours *unless the labeling specifically states otherwise.*

Culprit #2: Sugar

Sugar, just like refined flour, is an empty source of calories. Try to make every food choice count toward providing the nutrients you need. You are much better off eating foods that contain energy *plus* nutrients *and* fiber instead of empty calories. That doesn't mean you have to give up sugar entirely, just eat it in moderation.

Think about . . .
making good food choices

A good rule of thumb when choosing baked goods, cereals, crackers, pasta, muffins, waffles, pancakes and other high-carb foods is to check the label to make sure they contain at least 2 to 3 grams of fiber per 100 calories.

AVOID	INSTEAD
white baked goods	whole grains and whole-grain flours
cereals and crackers that contain hydrogenated or partially hydrogenated oils	choose cereals or crackers that are low in sugar and high in fiber
pasta made from enriched flour or enriched semolina	whole-wheat pasta; round out your meal with meat, cheese, veggies, and healthful, natural fats and oils
commercially prepared cookies, cakes and "sweet treats"	bake your own recipes using sugar substitutes

AVOID	INSTEAD
waffles and pancakes made from refined flour	eat whole-grain waffles and pancakes topped with cinnamon, nuts, ground flax seeds and fruits such as minced apples, sliced bananas and dried apricots
syrup and other sugary toppings	try thawed frozen berries, chopped nuts and nut butters; use real maple syrup or honey sparingly

Change How You Eat

Losing weight means more than simply changing what you eat. You also have to change HOW you eat. You need to slow mealtime down and eliminate the cues that lead you to eat when you're not really hungry.

To slow down your eating, try some of these strategies:

- ♥ Start your meal with a filling but lower-calorie food such as salad or a vegetable-based soup. At restaurants skip the appetizer, skip the bread, and start right up with the soup or salad.
- ♥ Take large sips of water between bites.
- ♥ Take smaller bites.
- ♥ Put less food on each forkful.
- ♥ Try to be the last person to finish a meal.

- ♥ Focus on the texture and flavor of your food. Dine on higher-quality food.
- ♥ Put your fork or food down between bites.

The Road to Self-Worth

One must eat to live, and not live to eat.

MOLIÈRE

I am the writer behind the scenes of a column for a national health and fitness magazine that focuses on success stories about weight loss. For years I have written about other people and their journey to a healthy body, mind and spirit. But I've never written my own success story. Sure, I've lost ninety-five pounds and have lowered my body fat from I don't even know how high to healthy, and dropped dress sizes from 24 to 10, but I always felt like that wasn't really me.

I wasn't always overweight. Until age five, I was a healthy, active kid. It wasn't until my parents started having problems that resulted in a divorce that I turned to food. I struggled with my weight all through my school years and into college, where I reached 260 pounds during my senior year. Today, more than a decade later, people don't believe that I ever weighed that much. Even I have to pull out the before pictures to remember, and they are shocking because back then I never looked in mirrors. I never looked other people in the eye for fear of what they would say about me. I was shy. I was ashamed. I was depressed. I was scared.

Like most of the people I interview for stories, I tried all the fad diets. My parents put me on them when I was a kid, and I forced myself on them as a teen and young adult. What I didn't realize was that the worst thing I could do was to use food as a form of punishment. It would never work. And it didn't.

One dark night before graduation, I looked at my body and imagined myself at eighty-five years old. If I continued walking the path I was on, who would I be? What would I look like? I saw overweight. I saw health problems. I saw loneliness and unresolved emotional pain. I didn't like what I saw. I remembered what an old college professor said to me when I asked her for advice. She merely shrugged and said, "You just have to choose."

I got mad at her. What kind of advice is that? Choose what? How can I choose? Then it clicked. It was a mental trick. All I had to do was choose the picture of who I wanted to be at eighty-five. All I had to do was choose to allow the real me to come out of her cocoon by making little choices in support of my decision every single day. I would deny myself nothing. I would choose to become the best me possible. I would choose health over habit. I would choose action over inertia. I would choose love over self-loathing.

I read the health books. I got educated. I learned balance. I went for walks. I chose to eat healthy and to not completely deny myself the things I loved, but I chose to eat them less often. And I chose to see it not as a short-term quick fix that would make me skinny tomorrow. I chose to see it as a lifelong journey to health. With the help of long walks and yoga, I learned how to listen to what my body wanted instead of the old tapes that made me crave sugar and junk food to numb out with.

It took a decade to lose that weight. I continue to lose a few pounds every year. I continue to listen to my body's needs. I know it needs sleep and downtime and play and inspiring work. I know that it needs good friends and healthy foods to fuel the things it wants to do. I know it needs movement and plenty of time outside.

Most of all I know that it needs gentle kindness and love from me. Not brutality. Losing weight over such a long time was like the proverbial herding of cats. Very gently, calmly and lovingly I would bring myself back to my goal of a healthy life each time I turned down a side road. I continue to gently shepherd my mind, body and spirit down my path to health. It's a road that I'll walk my entire life with love and gratitude because I am and have always been worthy.

♥ *Jacquelyn B. Fletcher*

Healthy Snacks

Here are some easy ways to start a healthy eating plan. Try at least two items from each list a week. Mix it up for variety. For lots more ideas, read my book, *The Gold Coast Cure*!

- **Vegetables.** For convenience, take advantage of precut raw vegetables and prepackaged salads. For dinner choose *either* fresh or frozen vegetables.

  ❑ broccoli

  ❑ spinach

  ❑ tomatoes

  ❑ asparagus

  ❑ green beans

  ❑ squash

  ❑ zucchini

  ❑ corn

  ❑ potatoes with the skins on

  ❑ sweet potatoes

  ❑ eggplant

- **Dips.**

  ❑ guacamole

  ❑ salsa

❏ tahini

❏ all-natural peanut butter

- **Fruit.** Buy either fresh fruit or frozen fruit.

  ❏ apples

  ❏ oranges

  ❏ grapes

  ❏ berries

  ❏ peaches

  ❏ raisins

  ❏ dried apricots

  ❏ dried plums

  ❏ dried mango

  ❏ dried pineapple

  ❏ dried apples

- **Cheese.** Purchase "light" or "low-fat" cheese for day-to-day use. Save full-fat cheese for gourmet meals on special occasions.

  ❏ feta

  ❏ low-fat shredded mozzarella

  ❏ fresh and shredded Parmesan and Romano

  ❏ goat cheese

  ❏ low-fat cottage cheese

- **Nuts and seeds.** Choose nuts and seeds that are either dry roasted or "raw." Don't be afraid of the calories in nuts. People who snack on nuts have been shown to weigh less than people who do not.

  ❑ peanuts

  ❑ walnuts

  ❑ macadamia nuts

  ❑ cashews

  ❑ almonds

  ❑ hazelnuts

  ❑ pecans

  ❑ sesame seeds

  ❑ sunflower seeds

  ❑ pumpkin seeds

Exotic Options

Make a pledge to try at least two of these healthy foods this week!

__**Old-fashioned oats.** Avoid refined "instant" oatmeal. Old-fashioned oatmeal cooks in about two minutes in your microwave. What could be easier?

__**Wheat bran and oat bran.** As a fiber booster add one tablespoon to the hot cereal of your choice. Each tablespoon contains two grams of filling fiber.

__**Wheat germ.** Add to your favorite hot cereal. Mix into breads, muffins and even cake.

__**Dried beans.** Cooking beans is as basic as cooking pasta and therefore beans make the perfect substitute. Be adventurous. Try black beans, black-eyed peas, cannelloni beans, garbanzo beans, great northern beans, Mexican beans, pinto beans, red kidney beans, lentils or green split peas.

__**Wild rice.** Try mixing wild rice with your regular rice.

__**Whole-wheat couscous.** Instead of white rice or pasta.

__**Whole-grain bread or whole-grain pita bread.** Instead of white bread or bagels.

Instead of eating _____

I'll try _____

Instead of eating _____

I'll try _____

Instead of eating _____

I'll try _____

Instead of eating _____

I'll try _____

A Sweet Good-Bye

We never repent of having eaten too little.

THOMAS JEFFERSON

From the time he was a little boy trading his peanut-butter sandwich for some other kid's raisins, my father has loved sweets. If it had sugar in it, he wanted it. At the age of thirty, though, all those little goodies were catching up with him. He had a pot belly and a few chins to match, so one day he gave up sweets entirely. He didn't cut back; he didn't try some fad diet, eating sweets only after five o'clock on alternate Thursdays. He simply said never again. No cookies hot from the oven, no gooey brownies, no crispy and crunchy caramel corn, no velvety creamy cheesecake, no tart but smooth key lime pie: all were banished from his mouth and his table. Not so much as an after-dinner mint would cross his lips.

People thought that he'd give up after a couple of months, but it's been thirty years now, and in all that time, he hasn't indulged in even a small bite of the Christmas fudge. He's been tempted by sugar-free goodies, but long ago he decided that one low-carb brownie would lead to the real thing, and in a month or two, he'd be eating chocolate-covered peanuts by the handful.

Instead of sugar, he started jogging. At first, he ran a couple of laps around the block, but in a couple of years, he was training for marathons. He went through blisters, sore knees, chafed skin and painful arches, but he kept running. He's now run marathons in a dozen states and a couple of foreign countries, and though he's cut back to half-marathons now that he's a granddad, he still thinks that a 10-kilometer race is like a day off.

These years haven't been easy for my father. My sister and I both love to bake, and I'm sure the sight of our chocolate pecan pies, lemon tarts and banana nut cake with cream cheese frosting (my specialty) left him salivating. No matter what temptation faced him, though, thinking of what he accomplished helped him to stay strong—or maybe watching my expanding rear end was deterrent enough.

My father's sister, on the other hand, never went in much for exercise or watching her diet. We live in the South, a place where even our pies are fried, and she's more than happy to indulge in all our regional treats. Whether it's fried chicken with pan gravy, creamy squash casserole or ham biscuits, her table (and every stomach nearby) is full to bursting with good things. Every holiday she whips up big batches of fudge, divinity and macaroons, and she definitely eats her share. The last time she ran, it was to the freezer to get some extra ice cream.

My father told her gently that maybe she should eat more vegetables and less sugar. "I've never touched that stuff, and I'm not going to start now," she'd say, piling up her plate with another serving of sweet-potato pie.

A couple of months ago, my aunt called my father. She had fallen victim to the family history of diabetes. She couldn't understand why my father had no signs of it yet, even though he was several years older.

My father thought of his years of eating salad and fish rather than Lane Cake and barbecue. He thought of those thousands of miles pounding the pavement rather than pushing the remote control. Then he just said that he guessed that he was just lucky. It wasn't time to say, "I told you so." He told her that it wasn't really so bad; if she watched her diet she could have many happy and healthy years ahead.

As soon as he got off the phone, he laced up his running shoes. He was going to make a happy and healthy future his own way.

♥ *Lydia Witherspoon*

Protein Tips

You can lose weight and have your meat, of course. Just try to follow these simple words of wisdom:

- **Chicken Hints.** Buy free-range chicken. Free-range chickens are fed healthy hormone-free diets and are left free to forage for much of their food. The result is a thinner, healthier chicken with superior flavor. All chickens store the majority of their fat just under their skin, so be sure to avoid eating the skin. White meat is better for you than dark meat.
- **Beef Hints.** Good cuts of beef include the round tip, top round, eye of round, top loin, tenderloin, filet mignon, sirloin and *extra-lean* ground beef. All-natural, hormone-free beef is your best choice. A serving of beef is about the size of your fingerless palm, not that enormous slab of beast served down at the local chop house.
- **Pork Hints.** The leanest cuts of pork include the tenderloin, top loin chop, center loin chop and loin roast. Trim all visible fat.
- **Fish Hints.** Aim for three to four servings of fish a week. On days you don't feel like cooking fish you can buy smoked salmon (lox), smoked

trout, canned salmon, sardines or canned tuna. Be sure to purchase canned fish packed in either water or olive oil. Avoid fish packed in soybean oil or any other type of processed vegetable oil. Avoid pre-breaded fish products.

- **Shellfish.** Also a great choice. Don't buy pre-breaded products.
- **Veggie Burgers.** Look for veggie burgers that don't have any hydrogenated or partially hydrogenated oil and contain at least 2 to 3 grams of fiber per 100 calories. And yes, they can be delicious.

My Page

My Thoughts _____

_____

_____

_____

My Feelings _____

_____

_____

_____

My Facts _____

_____

_____

_____

My Support _____

_____

_____

_____

Monday Morning Blues

*Tell me what you eat, and I shall tell you
what you are.*

ANTHELME BRILLAT-SAVARIN

My right hand dug deeper into the bag of chocolates, again! There I was, first thing Monday morning, breaking the promise I'd made the night before. I'd promised myself there'd be no more drowning my woes in a pound of chocolates or an entire loaf of hot crusty bread. But by mid-morning I'd consumed half of the bag of chocolates and had begun to devour a loaf of hot sourdough French bread, one slice after another, thickly spread with pure creamery butter.

It was amazing how I rationalized my behavior. I blamed it all on stress. After all, a large conglomerate had gobbled up my employer of twenty years, there'd been a reduction in salary and benefits, and I was subjected to longer work hours. And I continued to overindulge in food, which at the end of the day only made me fatter, not happier.

After six months of helping make the merger a smooth transition, I announced my retirement. After a magnificent retirement send-off, my husband and I purchased a condo where we'd always planned to retire, the central coast of California. Although I was retiring ten years earlier than planned, my husband assured me I had made the right decision. "You can finally do what you've always wanted to do, live near the ocean and write full-time."

I settled into the new community and made many new friends, most of them writers like myself. I thrived on being amongst my peers. I was overjoyed at the writing opportunities that came my way. Life was good. In the back of my mind lingered the nagging question; why was I still gorging myself with food? I even ignored my doctor's concern about my weight and reasons for lowering my cholesterol.

I was eating when I was glad and when I was sad; I was running out of excuses. I could no longer zip my favorite black slacks, and to my dismay they did not come in any larger size. That very Sunday evening I vowed to seek help on Monday morning. I'd follow my doctor's advice and sign up for weight counseling.

My knees shook when I approached the counter to register for weight counseling, but felt at ease when a gentleman with a smiling face greeted me, "Welcome, I'm one of the weight counselors here. My name is Frank."

I fought back the tears as I introduced myself and confessed to him how desperate I felt. As I filled out the paperwork, Frank uttered softly, "As of today, desperation and self-loathing are banished from your vocabulary."

Next, it was time to step on the scales. I didn't want to look, but I had to face the awful truth; I had gained forty pounds. I felt my cheeks grow hot, I closed my eyes, but that didn't stop the tears from trickling down my red face.

"You have to think of this as a lifestyle change, not a diet," Frank said, as he handed me a tissue. "This program is not a quick fix. Once you lose the weight you cannot go back to your old habits, and you won't want to."

My lifestyle change entailed banishing my two addictions, chocolate and white bread, from the house. Breakfast would no longer consist of choco-late candy and a cup of coffee. Actually, I'd forgot-ten I really liked cereal with fresh strawberries for breakfast.

The first week I lost three pounds. "So, during your first week did you have any problems getting used to eating healthy again?" Frank asked. I grumbled that keeping a journal of every morsel I put in my mouth was time consuming. Frank chuckled and replied, "When you nibble, you gotta scribble. It's the only way I've been able to keep my eighty pounds off for the past fifteen years."

I never complained again and faithfully wrote in my journal every day. I continued to lose weight, but it was a slow process. Frank's words kept me from getting discouraged. "Remember, set your goal weight at something you can live with. When you look at the weight range for your age, be realistic. Don't beat yourself up because you can't fit into the size you wore when you were a teenager."

I learned how to eat healthy; I was no longer a member of the clean-your-plate club. My exercise of choice was walking, and it worked. At the end of six months, I will never forget hearing Frank's exclamation, "Congratulations! You've lost 42.6 pounds! You've reached your goal!"

It has been two and a half years and I am still under my goal weight. I will admit there are days that I struggle, but food is no longer my security blanket. I've kept my promise, no more Monday morning blues for me!

♥ *Georgia A. Hubley*

Emotional Eating

One of the toughest challenges of losing weight is overcoming the urge to eat when you're *not* hungry.

If you're one of the many people who eat for emotional reasons, here's a solution: keep a food diary. Write down every single bite you put into your mouth, then write down exactly why you ate that bite of food. It works! The more you understand why you eat, the easier it will be to overcome overeating. For example, if you discover you nibble all day on snacks that add up to hundreds of extra calories because you're bored, you can come up with a game plan to prevent you from eating the next time boredom strikes.

Identify Those Harmful Emotions

The next time your emotions get the best of you and you're ready to grab the nearest danish, stop and think about what you're doing and why. Are you:

- **Angry?** Walk away from the situation that's making you boil over. Call a friend to commiserate.
- **Bored?** Go shopping, make plans to visit a friend, or do some reading. If you choose to shop, stay away from the mall with its food courts and fast-service restaurants!

- **Lonely?** Call a friend or make plans to join a class or club. Get involved in volunteer activities.
- **Anxious?** Turn off the news and turn on a comedy channel.
- **Sad?** Treat yourself to something special that doesn't involve food, like a movie or a facial. Exercising outdoors is a great way to boost your emotions when you're feeling low.

If your emotions are ruling your life, you may want to consider professional counseling. Sometimes it's best to deal with underlying depression or anxiety before starting your weight-loss program. Sometimes weight loss itself helps ease mild mood disorders. Ask for a referral to a licensed mental health professional such as a psychiatrist, psychologist or therapist from someone you trust, such as your family physician.

Is the Hunger Real?

Here are some ways to figure out if your hunger is physically or emotionally triggered:

- Emotional hunger comes on suddenly while physical hunger (so long as you avoid sugar and refined flour) comes on gradually.
- Emotional hunger feels like it needs to be fed immediately.

- Emotional hunger is more likely to produce food obsessions.
- Emotional eating won't stop when you're full.
- Emotional eating is more likely to produce feelings of guilt than after satisfying physical hunger.

⌛ Think about . . .
what to do when I'm bored

The next time I'm bored, I'll:

__ Drink a large glass of water or some other type of calorie-free drink.

__ Keep my hands busy by doing a puzzle or sending an e-mail.

__ Call a friend.

__ Weigh myself.

__ Take a walk.

__ Play with my child or pet.

__ Clean up a messy room.

__ Work in the garden.

__ Take a bubble bath.

To break the association you have between eating and many everyday activities, try some of these ideas:

- Take the light bulb out of your refrigerator.
- Don't eat at your desk.
- Don't eat in front of the TV or in your bedroom.
- Don't fill cookie jars or candy dishes.
- Use aluminum foil to wrap leftovers instead of plastic wrap so you won't be tempted by seeing what's inside.
- Freeze leftovers right away so you're not tempted to pick.
- Schedule a snack time during the day, then don't let yourself snack at other times.
- Don't shop when you're hungry. Avoid the bakery aisle.
- Make sure you sit when you eat.
- Never eat in your car.
- Change your routine so you don't walk by vending machines at work.

The Ultimate Steak Pie

If you wish to grow thinner, diminish your dinner.

HENRY SAMBROOKE LEIGH

Most of the time that Marion and Gary had been married, they had both been a bit on the heavy side. As the years passed, Gary took up golf and lawn bowling and his weight came down quite a bit. Marion was never sporty minded, and although in her early fifties she had piled on quite a few pounds, it didn't bother her until she got high blood pressure. That was when the doctor told her she would have to lose weight.

This made a real impact on Marion and she tried every possible way to lose weight, but without success. Although she and Gary constantly talked to each other as if they were enemies, their love for each other was really strong. Gary said that to help her he would eat whatever she ate and then she wouldn't be faced with temptation while cooking things for him.

He had no idea how little she ate on a diet and he

ended up starving! On his way back to work, he would buy supplementary food that he could eat without Marion knowing. It wasn't that he wanted to be deceitful, he just wanted to try to encourage her as much as he could.

Being a born and bred Scot, Gary's all-time favorite meal was steak pie. In Scotland, this is made with a rich, dark gravy full of onions, and covered in a rich puff pastry. In those days, the pastry was made with lard rather than any of the more modern-day healthy oils, so the calories in a steak pie were considerable!

Gary stuck with Marion's diet and she slowly began to lose weight. It was one Saturday when he was off to compete in a bowling tournament that he gave in to temptation with a vengeance. The main course at the hotel where the party was lunching was fish and chips, steak pie or a chicken salad.

Gary knew he should eat the chicken salad, but steak pie!!! He decided that since Marion would never know and he could go home and munch on the salad she would have for dinner that evening, it would be steak pie!

Since eating his favorite meal was now such a treat, Gary tore into it like a man who hadn't seen meat for weeks, and was finished in no time. A passing server looked at his empty plate, devoid of steak pie, pastry, potatoes, peas and carrots, and declared,

"Well, you must have been hungry!"

"I just love steak pie. My wife is on a diet, so we don't eat it at home just now!" he told her. Five minutes later back she came with another piece of steak pie and a few potatoes and peas. "We always do extra, and it would be a shame to waste it!" she said, putting it down in front of him.

Gary thanked her and found no difficulty at all in eating his second portion! By the end of it, he was too full to eat dessert, but he was happy.

They had eaten quite late as the tournament had run on a bit longer than planned so it was around 2:30 P.M. before they had their meal. They got into the bus and for once the roads were quite quiet. They got home by 5 P.M. Gary went into the house and shouted, "Hi Marion, I'm home!"

She came beaming at him from the kitchen, "I went for my weigh-in at the clinic this morning, and I have now lost eight pounds. Isn't that marvellous!" she asked.

He gave her a hug, absolutely delighted for her and was smiling happily until she said. "A lot of this is due to your help, Gary. I know how hard it must have been for you. When they told me how much I had lost, I stopped off at the butchers and bought some steak. As a 'thank-you' I have made a steak pie for your dinner!"

Gary stared at her and stammered, "Y . . . you have?"

"Yes, and it is all ready. You just go and sit down," she instructed.

Gary sat at the table and she put in front of him a huge plate of steak pie, mashed potatoes, peas and carrots!

He did his best to do it justice and make it look like it was the meal of a lifetime, so as not to disappoint her. When the phone rang and she went to answer it, he was delighted. He went into the kitchen cupboard, pulled out a plastic carrier bag and scooped some of the pie into it, and most of the peas and potatoes. As he heard her saying good-bye, he hurriedly dropped it into the kitchen garbage can and sat back down at the table.

He managed to eat some more of the meat and then sat back and confessed, "I am absolutely full, Marion, I couldn't manage another bite!"

She looked at the remains on his plate, something never known when Gary had steak pie and said, "You know, I think I can work out why you can't finish that!"

Gary's heart skipped a beat, until she said, "Since you've eaten the same as me for so long, your appetite has been reduced!"

♥ *Joyce Stark*

Weight Loss Is a Family Affair

You may be determined to lose weight, but that doesn't necessarily mean your family is interested in discovering new ways to eat. If you come from a family that values big, heavy meals, it may be difficult learning how to say "no" to that second helping. Your spouse and your children may not be so enthusiastic about your efforts to clear potato chips and cookies from the pantry. Don't get discouraged. They can adapt!

Dining Out

If your family is like most, you don't have time to prepare home-cooked meals every night. Eating out may well be a regular part of your meal plan. That's no excuse for not sticking to your new healthy way of eating! With a little creativity and some advance planning, you can almost always find a way to eat healthfully while dining out.

Remember, you don't have to clean your plate—some restaurants serve enormous portions! Other tips for dining out include:

- **Avoid the bread basket.** Those rolls are almost always made from refined flour, not whole grains. Restaurant sandwiches are not a good choice unless you skip the bread.

- **Order soups** containing beans and vegetables.
- **Eat salads, both as appetizers and as your entrée.** If you choose a salad as your main entrée be sure to add proteins such as chicken, fish and eggs, healthy fats such as low-fat cheese and avocado, and healthful fiber-rich good carbohydrates such as chick peas, beans and brown rice. Salads are one of your best restaurant picks because you can add so many healthy foods. Ask for your salad dressing on the side and stick to the vinaigrettes instead of creamy dressings. Order your salad without croutons, tortilla chips, and breaded meats or vegetables.

More Salad Tips:

- **Add vegetables.** The more vegetables the better! Try sliced tomatoes, cucumbers, shredded carrots, roasted squash, roasted red peppers, mushrooms, green beans or thinly sliced onions.
- **Add protein.** Steer clear of anything fried. Instead go for grilled chicken, grilled calamari, shrimp, seared tuna or even steak strips.
- **Add a small amount of cheese.** Keep cheese portions small unless the restaurant offers low-fat cheese. Most restaurant cheeses are rich in saturated fat. A little cheese adds a lot of flavor

and satisfaction to any salad. If there are no low-fat cheeses on the menu, standard parmesan is a good choice.

- **Add nuts, seeds, olives or avocado.** These good fats keep you feeling full and satisfied.
- **Add beans or corn**, two fiber-rich good carbohydrates that fill you up, not out!

Other restaurant suggestions:

- Choose foods that are steamed, broiled, baked or roasted, instead of fried.
- Select grilled seafood and grilled chicken instead of pasta, beef or fried foods.
- Share foods, such as a main dish or dessert, with your dining partner.
- Take part of the food home with you and refrigerate immediately. To make sure you have leftovers ask for a take-home container when the meal arrives. Put half the meal into this container so you're more likely to eat only what's left on your plate.
- Ask that your meal be served without gravy, sauces, butter or margarine. Olive oil, herbs and spices are more healthful alternatives.

Fast-Food Dilemma

Are the kids demanding dinner at their favorite fast-food restaurant? Just because you're determined to lose weight doesn't mean your family must never eat at a quick-serve restaurant again. Luckily, most fast-food restaurants now provide healthier options and nutrition information, so you can usually find something on the menu that won't throw a wrench into your eating plans. Some ideas for healthier eating:

- Ask for water, diet soda or skim milk instead of sodas and shakes.
- Order a grilled chicken sandwich without the sauce.
- Go bun-less!
- Order pizza with vegetable or chicken toppings instead of extra cheese. Don't eat the crust.
- Go easy on the cheese and steer clear of the tortilla chips when ordering Mexican. Add extra salsa and extra beans.
- Choose a salad instead of fries.
- Share! If you absolutely have to have some fries, don't eat an entire order yourself.

Think about . . .
the holiday eating trap

Oh, the holidays . . . family reunions, reminiscing, old family recipes for buttery cakes and pies—what's a healthy eater to do? Don't despair—you can get through the holidays without derailing your new nutritious eating plan. Before the holidays this year, choose which strategies will work best for you:

__ I will eat dried fruit, figs, nuts and dates instead of chocolates and sweets.

__ I will load up on fruit and vegetable side dishes so I'll be less likely to eat the high-calorie dishes.

__ When I'm baking, I'll use raisins or nuts instead of chocolate chips.

__ To make sure I don't binge at a holiday party, I'll eat small frequent meals during the day.

__ I will just make one visit to the buffet table!

__ If I have to try Aunt Bessie's cookies, I'll limit myself to just one.

__ I will limit drinking alcohol, since it will lead me to eat more.

__ I will find low-calorie, low-sugar, whole-grain recipes for traditional holiday foods such as stuffing or eggnog, or else I'll make two versions—traditional and healthy.

__ When I'm going to a party, I'll bring along a healthy item that I and other guests can enjoy, such as vegetables with a yogurt dip or reduced-fat cream cheese.

__ I will keep space between the food items on my plate to avoid overeating.

__ I will focus on maintaining my weight rather than weight loss during the holidays.

__ If I don't have time for my regular exercise routine during the holidays, at least I'll take a family stroll after a big meal.

__ When it's my turn to host the holiday meal, I'll send guests home with the higher-calorie, less healthy foods. Or I'll donate the leftovers to a shelter.

My Page

My Thoughts _____

_____

_____

_____

My Feelings _____

_____

_____

_____

My Facts _____

_____

_____

_____

My Support _____

_____

_____

_____

Just Listen to Mom

In the long run men hit only what they aim at.

HENRY DAVID THOREAU

Mrs. Shatzel outdid herself with this spelling assignment. She asked her students to each pick a classmate, write them a letter using all twenty words in the unit and mail it to their home.

Back in the 1960s, we sixth-graders used the phone and recesses in school to stay in touch. We didn't write letters, so this assignment was a really unique experience. I couldn't wait to receive my letter in the mail, running home each day to see what the carrier had delivered. And finally, one sunny April afternoon, it arrived. I tore open the envelope, unfolded the paper and gazed at the salutation.

It read, "Dear Lard Bucket."

I never forgot how I felt reading those words. Armed with plenty of motivation but little information, I embarked on a cycle of fast, binge and surrender, repeating the same mistakes throughout my adolescence into adulthood. The spirit was willing, but the brain wasn't quite engaged.

Last year I turned forty-five and had long since entered "surrender" mode when my friend Joe proposed a friendly wager: the first to lose 10 percent of his total weight would take the other and his wife out for dinner. What did I have to lose?

So Lard Bucket accepted the wager, halfheartedly. In return, Joe gave me a copy of a fitness profile he had received from a trainer, emphasizing that the recommendations were personalized to his condition. In reading the profile and recalling dozens of past failed attempts, I was overwhelmed by the possibilities. For this round of fast and binge, should I go low cal, high protein, low carb, low fat, gym rat, diet pills, food supplements, Hollywood Bimbo Grapefruit Diet, or try one of the million variations and combinations of all of them? Or maybe it would be better to just make the dinner reservations.

That's when The Pattern started taking shape. It was as if Mom was painting the big picture between the lines of detail in Joe's fitness profile. Everything fit. The profile said to eat many small meals in a day; Mom always said to eat only when you're hungry. The profile said to eat "x" thousand calories per day; Mom always said never to go hungry. The profile said people are hungriest in the morning; Mom always said to eat a good breakfast. The profile said

Joe should lose no more than two pounds per week; Mom always said to take the weight off slowly so you won't put it back on quickly.

Mom was right all along; it was only that her advice was too general to apply without information, and now I had that.

I went to work starting with the goal itself. Saying "I need to lose the weight of an average SUV by next summer" sets you up to fail. Saying "I will lose 1.5 to 2 pounds per week, *on average,* every week until I reach my desired weight" becomes a recipe for success and minimizes the likelihood of a binge on the rebound.

Since you can't get discouraged if you know what to expect, there was now no fear in weighing myself every day. Weight loss is an up-and-down process. As long as the weekly average was on target, I was fine.

It took almost a year, but I have shrunk from 243 pounds to 183, from a 44 waist to a 34, and have more energy and ambition than I ever dreamed possible. Best of all, I have the knowledge and understanding needed to keep the weight off, as I have done for almost a year. And it wasn't difficult at all. I just needed to listen to Mom.

♥ *James Hammill*

Avoid the Relapse Trap

Losing weight is only the first step toward achieving a healthier, fitter life. You also need to keep the weight off. That's where so many people fail. But if you come up with a plan to maintain your weight loss even *before* you've met your weight-loss goal, you'll find it a lot easier to keep yourself on track.

It's unrealistic to think you're never going to go on a food binge again. Give yourself permission to fail—occasionally—but work toward making failure happen less and less. While it's helpful to do advance planning for big occasions—such as deciding what you will and won't eat at your family reunion—all is not lost if you don't stick to your plan. Accept the fact that things might not go as you intended, and return to your new, healthy eating style once you get back home.

Maintaining Your Weight

To help maintain your new weight:

- Plan and shop for your weekly menu ahead of time.
- Eat all three meals every day plus a snack or two so you're not tempted to binge come late evening.

- Partake of only a little bit if you just have to taste a favorite treat, and make sure you don't overindulge the rest of the day.
- Decide ahead of time how you will handle being offered foods that aren't part of your new lifestyle. Practice turning them down—not rudely, but firmly.
- Keep a supply of healthy foods at home. Don't shop when you're hungry, and stick to your shopping list.
- Learn to eat slowly—drink lots of water during the meal, take little breaks while eating, and if you feel like you want seconds, wait about twenty minutes to see if you are really still hungry for those extra calories.
- Plan ahead! Decide before you go to a party or out to eat what you're going to have. Find out whether the restaurant offers a selection of healthy foods.
- Be choosy in what you eat. Eating at a friend's house or a buffet table doesn't entitle you to a free-for-all.
- Keep that exercise plan going strong. If you find yourself dragging, get an exercise partner or else sign up for a fun fitness class.
- Grab a piece of fruit or drink a glass of water, then GET OUT OF THE KITCHEN if you're hungry.

- Get out of the house if you feel like it's time to binge. Take a walk instead. Or call a friend.
- Choose one place in your house where you can eat—and don't let yourself eat anywhere else, including in front of the TV.
- Know what situations are likely to trigger lapses from your healthy eating plan, such as being lonely, bored or over-hungry. Develop a plan to cope with each of those situations in advance.
- Eat just a little bit if you absolutely have to indulge in a high-calorie food. If you don't, you're going to obsess about it until you end up eating the whole thing!

All Is Not Lost

If you do relapse into your old eating patterns, all is not lost. Don't let negative thinking allow you to toss all your hard-earned success away. Losing weight is not an all-or-nothing proposition. Relapsing isn't failing—you just have to get back in the swing of things. Getting mad at yourself won't help matters—instead, take positive steps quickly so it won't happen again. The important thing is to nip the problem in the bud, before five pounds become ten or twenty.

If you feel yourself relapsing:

- Get back into the swing of things—start exercising more, then cut back on snacks and sweets until your scale weight drops back down.
- Use a food diary to keep track of what you're really eating. Maybe you're starting to eat more than you intended to.
- Drink more water.
- Go back to the support group you once found helpful.
- Return to whatever strategies helped you lose weight in the first place.

Think about . . .
learning from past failures

Every time you've lost weight and regained it in the past, you've learned something—you've learned what doesn't work! Don't view relapses as failures. In fact, you've been testing different ways to keep the weight off all your life. At least now you know what not to try again.

To prevent weight gain, make a list of what has worked and what hasn't worked for you in your past attempts at losing weight. For instance, maybe you chose an exercise plan that wasn't realistic because you couldn't fit it into your routine, so you dropped it altogether. Maybe you forced yourself to give up a favorite food altogether instead of just cutting back to an occasional portion. Don't forget the things that did work, either—healthy foods you stocked up on or particular types of exercise that made you feel energized.

Strategies that worked for me when I lost weight in the past were:

1) _____

2) _____

3) _____

Strategies that didn't work:

1) _____

2) _____

3) _____

I'll Take Broccoli for 100, Alex

*Imprisoned in every fat man a thin one is wildly
signaling to be let out.*

—CYRIL CONNOLLY

W hen I was born, the nurses had to hold back
rolls of fat to clean me. It's an adorable image
for a newborn, but not exactly something you want
to carry around your whole life. All through my
youth I was fat, and in my mind I would always be
that way. I had to shop at special stores to buy pants
that would fit, and going to the pool was simply out
of the question. Who wants to see a flabby body like
mine? At one time or another, I had a nickname
related to nearly every kind of pastry in existence.
When they ran out of baked goods to compare me
to, they simply called me a bakery.

I had a desk job at a printing press when my
weight hit its peak. One morning I was driving to
work when I looked down at my stomach. It rolled
over my pants and spilled into my lap, looking like a
marshmallow-filled cloud that would not go away.

For the ten thousandth time in my life, I thought, *I'm sick of being fat. I'm going to lose weight.* It might as well have been a wish to travel to the moon. I was stuck in more ways than one, and my obesity seemed to be the most stubborn problem of them all.

A new gym was opening in town, but I ignored it. I told myself it was far too expensive, just in case I had considered marching through its doors. I was determined to stay in my slump, though needless to say I didn't really want to. Serendipity would have its way when I was called to my boss's office several days later. I left the room with a raise just large enough to pay for a gym membership. The moment of change was upon me. I knew I needed to act faster than I could make more excuses. I signed up that very afternoon.

It was the scariest place I had ever been. All those thin people with their tight clothes, trim bodies and non-flabby skin. I wanted to hide. But I had spent money, so I couldn't back down now. I was going to do this even if it embarrassed me beyond recognition. I avoided the thin people by working out early in the morning before the sun had risen. I had no routine and very little knowledge of how to do whatever it was I was supposed to do. I ran, lifted weights and watched *Jeopardy* while on the elliptical trainer. I even enlisted a friend to join me. We would run laps, counting in a different language

each day. Exercise is for nerds, too.

With my new gym membership came a spurt of action in my life. I began shaping up my diet, realizing exercise would only get me so far. Little Debbie snack cakes, once a staple of my diet, were replaced with vegetables and fruits. Portions were cut back, and I taught myself to cook some delicious meals. It was much easier than I thought, and I didn't miss my old ways one bit. Each day as the scale loomed below my feet, I would see the needle stop a little sooner. I was losing weight, slowly accomplishing my dream, and I was having a blast doing it.

My coworkers were amazed. Often they would come up to me and compliment my efforts, then lean in with a covert look in their eyes and whisper, "What's your secret?" I would grin, look side to side and reply, "Don't tell anyone, but I eat good food and exercise every day."

After a year of delightful meals and a lot of fun at the gym, I lost over 100 pounds. That's almost a full person trimmed from beneath my skin. Twelve inches had vanished from my waist, permitting me to shop anywhere I pleased. No one calls me jellyroll anymore, and when I walk down the street I don't feel eyes glued to my stomach in disgust. I feel light in body and light in heart, all thanks to a few vegetables and goofing off at the gym.

♥ *John Bardinelli*

Trading Fat Cells for Barbells

She whips out her appointment book and cheerfully rattles off open times. "First thing in the morning is always good." She lies.

Nothing is good first thing in the morning except coffee in bed. In fact, the best thing first thing in the morning *is* my bed.

"What about 5 A.M. or 10?" Dancing brown eyes shimmer over a smile that cuts her face in half. She is all teeth and joy. Even her name is cheerful— Lorri Ann. I had hoped for someone as somber about this situation as I. If fitness centers are great places to meet people, I wanted someone I could relate to right off the bat. Someone who knows that this is the last stop on the road to the end of the world. At least the world as I knew it.

"Weight training is so exciting. You won't believe how it will make you feel. We can reshape your body like PLAY-DOH. When you come in, first thing we'll do is fat testing. Then we'll measure your dimensions."

I was never keen on tests in school. My fat did

not wiggle for joy upon notice that it too would endure a test of its own.

Her enthusiasm ricocheted off a 40-foot ceiling. "You're really gonna love it." She lied again.

Cautiously, I returned to the gigantic lobby of the big, fancy health facility (BFHF) early one Friday. Thawing out under the bright lights of the BFHF I pondered the lighting. Brightness burst through big windows and down from the ceiling like those merciless bulbs in dressing rooms that highlight your figure flaws when you are at your most vulnerable—trying on clothes.

"I'm so glad you're here, Suzan!" Lorri Ann Code bounced towards me with that beaming face of hers.

Health clubs make me feel uneasy. Over the years I have entered their doors after occasional bouts of bottoming out from my lifestyle of denial, indulgence, denial, indulgence, repeat. These clubs attract spandex-laden lassies with perky ponytails who strut in glittery tights. I wear old maternity pants just to get through the buffet line during the holidays.

"Let's begin!"

I filled out health history forms then, with Lorri Ann, and established "measurable goals." It was important that I understand what I wanted out of this undertaking.

I wanted it to be over.

I also wanted stronger bones and tighter everything else. I knew that New Year's resolutions often fail because we promise on the heads of our children to give up something without considering that we are actually taking on a *lifestyle change.* Clearly, bowing out of this commitment would be difficult with Captain Code around. Accountability this time had a face with a big grin on it.

We headed for the equipment—gigantic conglomerations of metal with pulleys and cables connected to an array of weights. Captain Code demonstrated each apparatus, which strengthen and tone different muscles. I followed her lead, receiving encouraging remarks and gentle corrections, "Keep your wrists straight, put your head back, align your back, don't rotate your shoulders." She wrote copious notes on my workout sheet denoting the number of repetitions, weight used, posture, seat height, where my feet go and so forth.

Code does not tolerate a sloppy performance. "You'll get great benefits, but you have to use the machines correctly. When you come back next time, you'll go first and I'll tell you what you are doing right and what you are doing wrong. It's the best way to learn."

I can hardly believe I am finally keeping a promise I'd made for fifteen years—to learn weight training.

"The first four weeks we build a base," she says. "After that, we'll develop a program where you can work your upper body one day, lower another, or do a combination. Does it hurt yet?" She smiles. "Four more, three, two, one, rest and stretch for sixty seconds. Do you mind being sore in the morning? Wait until tomorrow night!"

I claim I don't mind pain later, but in the heat of the moment I am adverse to it. She says something else but I don't hear it, distracted by a man with arms the size of the Sierra Nevada Mountains. The next fifteen reps whip by. Some views in the BFHF are not designed to go unnoticed. People of all ages and sizes are there. A variety of "before, during and afters," I consider. It is comforting to see folks in their thirties, forties and fifties. I thought mostly twenty-year-old blondes in tights went to health clubs. At forty-five, I was in the right demographic in my Big Dog gym pants.

We concluded with a cardiovascular workout. Captain Code gave me a choice of stair steppers, exercise bikes, treadmills and other pieces of equipment designed with your sweat in mind. "You'll start to burn fat after twenty minutes."

"Put the timer on thirty," I bravely retort.

"Good girl! You're doing great!" She says this for the twentieth time. I love hearing it. An hour of being the center of attention when I am used to ignoring my needs in lieu of family demands felt surprisingly rejuvenating. I wanted more.

Lorri Ann whipped out a set of headphones called "Cardio-Theater" and plugged them into a box on the machine. Two television sets hang from the ceiling in front of us. "This TV is Channel 4, that one is Channel 15, or you can listen to music or talk shows."

Working out wasn't so bad after all. The handle of my treadmill measured my heart rate. I felt sudden exhilaration. I had a trainer! At long last I was learning the correct way to use intimating equipment that would tone my body in new and unexpected ways. And perhaps my attitude might get toned in the process. For the first time in ages, I felt like a star.

❤ *Suzan Davis*

Exercise—Getting Started

You don't look good in sweats; you're not coordinated; you're out of shape. . . . It's not difficult to come up with 100 reasons not to exercise. The truth is all you need to do is set aside a little time. Even ten minutes three times a week is a good start—you can work your way up to thirty minutes as your stamina improves. You don't even have to leave the house—exercising with a video in front of your TV in the privacy of your own home is just as effective as exercising outdoors or exercising at the gym.

Exercise Choices

- **Walking** is a great way to get started, especially if you haven't exercised much before. At first, don't worry about how quickly you walk. To build muscle and speed your weight loss, try walking with light handheld weights. If you're concerned walking will put stress on your back, hips or knees, you may want to try walking in a pool.
- **Cycling,** either on a real bicycle or on a stationary machine, provides a good aerobic workout. For best results try riding up and down gentle hills. Be sure you dial up at least some resistance on stationary machines.
- **Aerobic dance** is a great way to get fit and meet

new people. Many aerobic classes incorporate weight training into their routines. Low-impact aerobics, in which one foot is always on the ground (no jumping or running in place), is safer, especially if you're new to exercise or more than a little bit overweight. Try beginners' aerobic dance videos, too.

- **Swimming** exercises your whole body and won't overstress your muscles and joints. Pushing the water away from you provides natural resistance that builds up your muscles. You can add to the resistance effect by using handheld paddles.

- **Circuit training** with weight machines is a highly effective technique available in most gyms. You can also circuit train with dumbbells in the privacy of your own home. Try to work out with weights at least twice a week if at all possible. We highly recommend weight training as part of our *Gold Coast Cure* to boost metabolism and help you drop clothing sizes.

Here are some other ideas to get you started:

- Choose activities you enjoy and can fit into your daily schedule. Don't choose a morning swim routine if you hate getting up early.

- Don't worry if you miss a day or two—just do your best to make exercise a regular part of your life. Soon you'll realize you don't feel quite so good when you don't exercise!

- Find someone who will exercise with you.

Choosing a Gym

If you're the type of person who finds it motivating to exercise in a group, you'll want to look into joining a gym, the local Y, or a hospital-affiliated wellness program. You don't have to spend a lot of money to find a nice, clean place to exercise—many communities have low-cost community centers offering a gym and workout classes. Don't choose a facility that's too far away—you may be motivated to go now, but will you still want to drive there three times a week next winter? Is the facility's schedule convenient for you? Make your initial visit at the time of day you're most likely to go when you're a member. See whether there's a long wait for the equipment you want to use. Make sure there are classes geared to your ability level. Are there staff members available to show you how to correctly use the equipment?

Get a Nutritious Start

Just like your car needs fuel to drive, your body needs fuel to exercise. Here are some tips to get you started:

- Always eat a breakfast that includes filling whole

grains, cereals and fruits. This is important even on the days you are not exercising.

- Ideally, several hours before you work out, eat a balanced meal containing carbohydrates, fats and protein—such as whole-grain bread with sliced turkey, condiments and 2 percent milk, or an all-natural peanut butter sandwich on whole-grain bread accompanied by a salad topped with olive oil vinaigrette or yogurt, or a whole-wheat pasta dish topped with tomato sauce and lean ground meat.

- If you aren't able to plan that far ahead, snack on foods half an hour or so ahead of time that are lower in fat and easily digested, so that you have enough energy for your workout—good choices would be fruit; high-fiber, all-natural crackers; low-fat cottage cheese; skim milk; or a small turkey breast sandwich on whole-grain bread.

- Always drink plenty of water before, during and after your workout to prevent your muscles from becoming cramped or sore.

Ask Your Doctor

Be sure to consult with your doctor before starting an exercise program if any of the following apply:

- You are a man over forty or a woman over fifty

- You have a heart condition
- You feel discomfort in your chest when you do physical activity
- You ever become dizzy or lose your balance
- You have a bone or joint problem
- You are diabetic
- You take blood pressure or heart medications

Even if your doctor gives you the green light, it is probably safer to exercise at a hospital-sponsored wellness center if you have a history of recent heart problems. Do not let health problems keep you out of the gym altogether!

Think about . . .
my favorite exercise

List these activities on a scale of 1 to 5, with 5 being the most desirable. If you don't see your favorite exercises here, add them in the space below.

_____ Aerobics
_____ Basketball
_____ Bicycling
_____ Dancing
_____ Golf
_____ Hiking
_____ Jogging
_____ Soccer
_____ Swimming
_____ Tennis
_____ Walking
_____ Weights
_____ Yoga

My goal is to:

Get exercise through _____ at least _____ times a week for _____ minutes each time.

WEEKLY EXERCISE CHART

	Time	**Activity/Exercise**	**Minutes**
Monday			
Tuesday			
Wednesday			
Thursday			
Friday			
Saturday			
Sunday			

The Green Giant of Fitness

Age is strictly a case of mind over matter. If you
don't mind, it doesn't matter.

JACK BENNY

My knees were shot. The X-rays didn't show cartilage damage, which might have been repaired the easy way, with surgery. Mine had wear and tear from carrying too much weight for too long.

For months, I wrestled with the decision of how to make changes, eating myself up another twenty pounds until I knew for sure I had to at least attempt to get a grip. Like so many others, I had already been on a million diets and lost hundreds of pounds, only to gain them back plus more. It seemed like my problem was more in my head than in my stomach, so when I saw the advertisement for a hypnotist, I decided to fork over the forty-nine bucks to try and get my head straight.

We sat there, a room full of pudgies, some pudgier than others, some so thin that those of us with a lot to lose wondered why they were even there. I soon learned that often size and feeling out of control are a state of mind. Just because some weren't huge didn't mean they felt in control.

I don't know why this time felt different, but what the guy was saying to us made sense. He didn't expect us to cut down to forty calories a day, or hang from a doorway, or measure our meals in a thimble, or run the Alps. He encouraged us to go at it a little at a time.

"When I first began I could barely walk to my mailbox without panting," he said.

Sounds like me! Was I ready? Like an alcoholic in recovery I decided to try one day at a time. I'd be more conscious of what I was eating, eat slower, try not to put too much on my plate, drink water and never, ever beat myself up if I felt I'd made a bad choice. Most important, I would not step on a scale for at least a year . . . maybe longer . . . maybe never! If the scale is my enemy, then why do I let it dictate to me?

I bought the tapes and vitamins and wondered if I had been duped by a charlatan. Two days later I begged my husband to go for a walk in the park with me. I barely made it around the small circle, limping like a linebacker after the big game and dragging one leg behind me like the Hunchback of Notre Dame. I listened to the tape faithfully for three months, but didn't really do as much exercise as the tape told me I should. It's okay. I still did more than I had ever done before. NO beating myself up for feeling inadequate!

I walked more and even joined a water-aerobics class. I hurt and ached through the whole thing, wondering if I was doing more damage than good. I kept four bags of frozen peas in the freezer to ice my joints after exercise . . . sometimes a knee, sometimes two, maybe my back, a shoulder, even an elbow a few times. I was the Green Giant of fitness!

The pool exercise was great because it afforded me flexibility and stamina I didn't have on land. Still, at the end of a session, I couldn't grab my ankle to do the runner's stretch so I leaned against the wall. I couldn't walk far so I took short walks more often. I made adjustments for me, worked at my pace, no one else's.

Three months passed. I used the tape less and less. Six months. I didn't seem to go as nuts as I used to; yet when I felt myself dropping over the edge, faced with a whole barrel full of Halloween candy, I'd put on the tape. If I still wanted one piece or even two when the tape was over, I'd eat them. Without guilt. NO beating myself up!

I don't know how many pounds dropped off and I really don't care. Most of my clothes are simply too big to even think of wearing, so it's probably a substantial number. A year later, to celebrate not going off the deep end too often, I thought of weighing myself. No, that's still not for me. Instead, I successfully grabbed my ankle to do the runners stretch.

One gorgeous, perfect fall day, I decided I'd take a walk . . . around a lake . . . six miles. It took me three hours. I might never do it again. I don't care. I did it! And when I was finished I was tired, but I didn't even need one bag of frozen peas!

♥ *Mary Mooney*

Finding Support

While it is important that you lose weight for yourself, seeking support from others can make your job easier. You'll have to figure out which people in your life will be the ones to encourage you and not sabotage your efforts. Choose people who will listen to you, exercise with you, and share your interest in healthy eating.

Picking a Support Person

A good support person can be, but isn't always, someone you live with or see every day. Not every spouse, sibling or best friend is a great person to help you overcome your challenges as you lose weight. You don't want to choose someone who says critical things about you and your weight, and you certainly don't want to pick someone who pushes food on you. Stay away from people who are competitive with you and people who don't understand or won't take the time to try to understand how difficult it can be to lose weight.

Is a Support Group Right for You?

- Do you like being part of a group?
- Do you like to talk about your feelings with others?
- Do you want to hear stories about other people and their weight-loss experiences?

- Are you looking for helpful hints or do you want to share your advice with others?
- Would such a group make you feel better?

There is no reason to feel guilty about taking advice from a group of strangers rather than your family and friends. The number-one reason people join a support group is to be with other people who have "been there"—not because of lack of support from friends and family.

Meet in Cyberspace

Not only do support groups meet in person, there are also many successful online chat rooms and online support networks geared toward weight loss. These Internet support groups can be a big help if you prefer the privacy of an electronic identity. With Internet groups, you can seek support at any time of the day or night.

While electronic therapy can provide valuable emotional support, chat rooms may not always offer correct medical information. Be careful about any health information you get from the Internet. Use caution when comparing stories and treatments. What's right for someone else may not be right for you. Check with your doctor before making any dietary or activity changes based upon Internet hearsay.

⧖ *Think about . . .*
choosing a support person

When choosing a support person, look for someone who has as many of the following qualities as
possible. Check off all that apply to the person
you've chosen. If you don't check off at least four,
consider finding a different support person:

My support person:

__ Makes me feel comfortable when we discuss
my weight.

__ Is likely to be sympathetic to the challenges I
will encounter as I try to lose weight.

__ Compliments me and makes reassuring
comments.

__ Is available when I need him or her.

__ Tends to offer good advice.

My Page

My Thoughts _____

_____

_____

_____

My Feelings _____

_____

_____

_____

My Facts _____

_____

_____

_____

My Support _____

_____

_____

_____

What's the Point?

I can resist everything except temptation.

—OSCAR WILDE

The women in my family have been living by a number system for the past several weeks, so the other day I decided to get in on the program too. This program now assigns every edible item on the face of the earth a corresponding point value, and according to your present weight, you get a pre-set number of points (or food) that you can eat. Therefore, if you're lucky, that means you can have three meals a day . . . as long as you don't mind gum for one of them. The points add up quick. For example, a slice of bread is two points. An enchilada is nine points, and a meal at McDonald's is one million, two hundred and twenty-nine thousand, seven hundred and eighty-nine points—or better yet, your last meal on Earth.

The night before my diet was set to start, I checked out the chart to see how many points I could eat each day. Based on my weight, I'm allowed twenty-five. Seeing that wouldn't work for me, I decided that because I'm a man, and therefore I have the role of hunter-gatherer in the family, I should have extra points. So I gave myself thirty points a day. In other words, I added up the equivalent of twenty-five points and realized that if I stuck to that meager plan, I wouldn't be able to operate heavy machinery. But don't think that extra five points buys me a trip down the buffet line. There are only degrees of starvation.

Actually, I did think that the first day went fairly smoothly—mostly, I guess, because the night before the diet, I binged as a farewell to my old eating habits and woke up the next day barely able to walk. Still, by evening, I was starving. So my wife asked me how many points I had left for dinner. I rolled my eyes. "I have enough to enjoy a tablespoon of dirt," I answered, "as long as there aren't any bugs (five points) in it . . . or mulch (nine points)." The diet has gone downhill from there. To be successful, you really have to learn how to space your points out evenly throughout the day. That way, by dinnertime, you still have enough so you don't get a hunger headache, or your stomach doesn't rumble and frighten small children.

There's a discipline to the program, which, incidentally, my wife is really good at following. Just yesterday morning she was bragging about it. "I banked three points yesterday," she announced.

I looked up from licking the bottom of my cereal bowl. "What does that mean?"

"I didn't use three points," she exclaimed.

I wanted to cry. "I'll give you ten dollars for them."

"You can't buy MY points," she answered.

"Why not?" I argued. "You're not using them."

"Yes, I am," she retorted. "I can apply them to my points today—I'm going to have a latte with my lunch."

"Yum," I said. "I'll give you five dollars to smell your breath." I think I might have to up my daily points—like maybe by one million, two hundred and twenty-nine thousand, seven hundred and eighty-nine.

♥ *Ken Swarner*

Commercial Weight-Loss Programs

Some people do better following the more structured approach offered by commercial weight-loss programs. Before you sign up for any weight-loss program, here's what the National Heart, Lung, and Blood Institute recommends you ask:

- **Does the program provide counseling to help you change your eating activity and personal habits?** The program should be geared toward teaching you how to make permanent changes to your diet and lifestyle. Plans designed to last a specific number of days, weeks or months are less effective.

- **Is the staff made up of a variety of qualified counselors and health professionals such as nutritionists, registered dietitians, doctors, nurses, psychologists and exercise physiologists?** If you have any health problems, take medicine, or you want to lose more than about 15 to 20 pounds, you need to be evaluated by a physician.

- **Is training available on how to deal with times when you may feel stressed and slip back to old habits?** The program should provide long-term strategies to deal with the weight maintenance problems you may have in the future. Having an ongoing support system in place that you can take advantage of at any time is important.

- **Is attention paid to keeping the weight off? How long is this phase?** Find a program that will show you how to make permanent changes in eating and activity levels to prevent weight gain.
- **Are food choices flexible and suitable? Are weight-loss goals set by the client and the health professional working together as a team?** Individual food preferences and individual lifestyle necessities should be taken into account when weight-loss goals and strategies are planned and discussed.

Other important questions to ask:

- What percentage of people complete the program?
- What is the average weight loss among people who finish the program?
- What percentage of people have problems or side effects? What are they?
- Are there fees or costs for additional items such as special foods and dietary supplements?
- Does the program make claims that are just too good to be true, like easy weight loss, rapid weight loss or a lifetime guarantee?

The Secret

For years I searched for "The Secret" to weight loss. If I found "The Secret," then I could pass it on to my daughter and be able to share it with the world. She and I have lost a little more than fifty pounds each. Together we've lost the equivalent of one of those little Olympic gymnasts we saw on TV. We found "The Secret."

My daughter is a wonderful example of the correct way to lose weight. She looked in the mirror one day and said to herself, *I like who I've become and what I've done with my life. I don't like the way I look; I think I'll do something about it.* She found what suited her: help on the Internet. The online source for weight-loss support helped her to establish guidelines for food intake and exercise, and also offered a support group for tips and advice. She stayed within the calorie, carb and fat counts outlined for her. She joined a gym and faithfully exercised three to five times a week. From April to October she steadily lost weight, going from a size 18W to a 10 Misses. Her confidence and self-esteem zoomed through the roof.

I started last fall on what I had hoped would be my final effort to lose weight. Unfortunately, I wasn't very successful. Health problems and medications, especially the amount of insulin I was taking for diabetes, hindered my success. I finally started researching weight-loss surgery. I found a lot of information on the Internet, talked to people I knew who had the surgery and started telling others what I was considering. People knew people who had had the surgery. I learned that weight-loss surgery is not a magic bullet, but is another tool to use in a comprehensive weight-loss program. Three months ago, I decided to go for it.

I am fifty-six years old and have had problems with compulsive overeating all my adult life. My struggles with weight loss started at age six when I observed my older sister and aunt suffering as they tried to lose weight. I decided then that I never wanted to diet. When I was ten, my new stepmother let me know I was fat, and dieting became a constant in my life. Even as a teenager, when I swam and water-skied all the time, my father and stepmother kept after me to just not eat and to slim down. But nobody ever really helped me choose good foods or change my eating habits. Eventually every effort failed.

As an adult I regularly pursued whatever fad diet was popular at that time. I'd do what many do, the yo-yo thing, lose some, go off the diet, gain back more. Finally I decided to get serious help from doctors, therapists, nutritionists and God. With them in my corner, I was able to change some long-standing habits. I quit eating compulsively whenever I was feeling hurt, angry, happy or sad. I identified the roots of my feelings and learned to deal with emotions without food. The surgery has been a tool to help me complete the process. It has taken many years to get to this place. I still have 120 pounds to go to reach my goal weight. My energy level is way up; my use of medications is way down. I have gained what it takes to be successful at weight loss.

My daughter and I each, in our own way, have found "The Secret" to weight loss. "The Secret" is doing what works for you.

I would recommend her way first. Her way is the better way. My way works when diet efforts don't work—but I still have to work to reach my goal. That is why I know we will succeed and the weight will stay off: because we were, each in our own way, ready.

I have every confidence that with God's help and guidance we will both reach and maintain our goals. We are far too happy with today's results not to succeed.

♥ *Marilyn Eudaly*

The Last Resort:
Weight-Loss Surgery

Although most people can lose weight through healthy eating and exercise, some people seem destined to fail no matter how hard they try. The medical community does offer one effective, although radical, solution—weight-loss surgery. In experienced hands, weight-loss surgery is a medically appropriate last resort.

The ideal candidate

- has failed to respond to multiple medically supervised attempts at less radical weight-loss treatment and is still healthy enough to tolerate major surgery;
- is one hundred pounds or more above his or her ideal body weight;
- has a body mass index (BMI) between 35 and 40 *and* suffers from at least one major medical problem caused by obesity, such as diabetes or sleep apnea;
- has a BMI of over 40 without necessarily suffering from any other medical condition.

To figure out your BMI, use the BMI calculator at: *www.consumer.gov/weightloss/bmi.htm.*

All of the most commonly performed weight-loss surgeries work primarily by creating a very small stomach pouch that is easily stretched by small amounts of food. This results in a sensation of fullness that causes patients to eat less. The two most commonly performed weight-loss surgeries involve either stapling across the stomach (gastric bypass) or placing an adjustable silicone ring around a portion of the stomach (gastric banding).

Candidates for weight-loss surgery are typically referred by their primary care doctors to a weight loss (bariatric) surgeon. The American Society of Bariatric Surgeons (*www.asbs.org*) makes a listing of its membership available for the public to view. Regular members are all surgeons who performed at least twenty-five weight-loss operations in the two years prior to being initiated. Surgical experience is critical to the success of these operations.

There are a number of things to consider when deciding whether to pursue weight-loss surgery.

The Benefits:

- After surgery most patients lose weight quickly and continue to lose weight for 12 to 24 months. Many patients regain 5 to 10 percent of the weight they lose, but it is not uncommon to maintain a greater-than-100-pound weight loss.
- Most people who undergo weight-loss surgery

see marked improvements in their obesity-related medical problems such as diabetes, high blood pressure and sleep apnea.

The Risks:

- Between 10 and 20 percent of patients who have weight-loss surgery need more surgery to correct complications.
- Nearly one-third of patients who have weight-loss surgery develop nutritional deficiencies. These deficiencies can result in anemia, hair loss, osteoporosis and even nerve problems. Fortunately, nutritional deficiencies can generally be avoided by taking vitamin and mineral supplements and keeping up with regular medical follow-up.
- The surgery is very expensive, costing about $25,000. Medical insurance coverage varies widely by state and by insurance provider.

It's important to remember weight-loss surgery alone doesn't guarantee successful long-term weight loss. Success is only possible in patients who agree to cooperate fully with their doctor's orders, commit to lifestyle change, and obtain medical follow-up for the rest of their lives.

Bite Me: Or, a Funny Thing Happened on the Way to the Buffet Table

I love buffets. I can pick and choose exactly what to eat, and I'm expected to go back for seconds. And thirds. Maybe even fourths. The extra helpings are factored into the cost and, as a careful consumer, I want to get my money's worth.

So, when I lined up at a Chinese buffet, I knew exactly what to do. I straightened my back, squared my shoulders and got ready to scrimmage. Ignoring the soups and salads that are for amateurs, I headed right for the main dishes. Within minutes, my plate was filled with spare ribs, meatballs, duck, squid, grilled steak and Szechuan noodles. A large helping of carrots and broccoli topped off the extravaganza.

Staggering under my load, I returned to my table all set to dig in. I grabbed my fork and started eating. The first few bites were delicious as I sampled each delicacy in turn. The meat was tender, the sauces flavorful, the noodles nice and spicy, and the veggies crunchy. I was in buffet heaven.

The next few bites were also good. If the flavors

seemed a little less appetizing, I didn't let that get in the way of my enjoyment. I was into a rhythm: Fork, plate, mouth, chew, sigh with pleasure and then repeat.

Halfway through, a startling transformation occurred. My sigh shifted to a groan. I had moved from pleasure to satiation, and I still had half a pyramid of food left to eat. Well, I wasn't going to let anything as simple as feeling full stop me from eating.

I stuck my fork into a piece of steak smothered in teriyaki sauce and brought it to my mouth. But my mouth refused to cooperate and stayed stubbornly shut. As a buffet pro, I knew that wasn't supposed to happen until the fourth plateful of food. I gently waved the steak under my nose, letting the aroma waft upwards. Nothing. My lips were glued shut.

I put the fork down and took a minute or two to think about this new development. A waiter, seeing my half-full plate, rushed over to see if everything was okay. I nodded absently. As I sat there quietly, I began to feel a strange sensation in my stomach—a sensation of fullness. Not my normal "stretched to the limit I'm going to explode in a minute if I eat another bite" fullness but rather a "this is nice and I don't think I need any more" fullness.

I hadn't even hit the dessert table yet.

My first reaction was to demand my money

back. If I couldn't even finish one helping of food, there was obviously something wrong with the buffet. My second reaction was to smile. There was nothing wrong with the food; there was something right with me.

Three months of exercise and sensible eating had paid off. The connection in my brain between "buffet" and "overeat" had been short-circuited. Rather than wolf down everything in sight, I need only try a few bites of my favorite foods to be content. While the restaurant's profits might go up, the numbers on my scale didn't have to.

I walked out of the restaurant with my head held high and my pants still comfortably buttoned. And one almond cookie in my purse—for later.

♥ *Harriet Cooper*

Introducing . . . The New You!

When you've achieved your hard-earned goal—a thinner, healthier you—you're likely to find your life will change. Most of the changes will be positive, but some will surprise you—and some might take a little getting used to.

- **You'll be healthier.** People with Type II diabetes often find their disease is cured by weight loss. You can lower your blood pressure and your cholesterol level and even reduce your risk of heart disease and cancer with weight loss too.
- **Your energy level will improve.** You're likely to be more active for longer periods of time.
- **You'll have the opportunity to buy new styles and sizes of clothing.** For most people this is a welcome, fun opportunity but it can be scary, too, to realize it really is a new you in that dressing room.
- **Your confidence will get a boost, too.** While losing weight won't solve all your problems, you may feel better able to deal with them.
- **You can move on with your life.** Yes, you'll still have to devote time and energy to keeping your weight off, but you'll no longer have to make weight loss the center of your universe.

Changes that may take some getting used to include:

- **People may start to treat you differently.** They may have different expectations for the newly thin you that they didn't have when you were heavier. In the workplace, this can be a positive change. Some people report their bosses and colleagues see them as being more professional and disciplined once they've lost weight.
- **People of the opposite sex may start treating you differently.** This, too, may be a welcome change, but suddenly attracting attention after years of hiding behind your weight can be a bit unnerving. Attention may make you feel uncomfortable, at first, but you'll get used to it.
- **Friends and relatives who are still heavy may resent you.** They may even try to interfere with your efforts to maintain your new weight. They may disparage your lifestyle plan. You may even find yourself gradually turning toward a different set of friends for support.

No matter how different your life may seem once you've lost weight, remember, you're still you—only more confident, healthier and happier.

Think about . . .
positive changes in my life

The changes in my life I'm most looking forward to when I lose weight are:

Health

1)

2)

3)

Fashion/Appearance

1)

2)

3)

Social

1)

2)

3)

Attitude

1)

2)

3)

Resources

American Council on Exercise provides health and fitness information, including tips on exercise and free recipes. Contact them at:

4851 Paramount Drive
San Diego, CA 92123
Phone: 858-279-8227 or 800-825-3636
www.acefitness.org

American Dietetic Association provides nutrition information and helps consumers find dieticians in their local area. Contact them at:

216 West Jackson Boulevard
Chicago, IL 60606
800-877-1600, or 800-366-1655 for recorded food/
nutrition messages
www.eatright.org

American Obesity Association provides information on protecting yourself against weight-loss fraud. Contact them at:

1250 24th St., NW, Suite 300
Washington, DC 20037
800-98OBESE
www.obesity.org

American Society of Bariatric Physicians (ASBP) offers information on the growing problem of obesity, tips on weight loss, and a referral program to reach their member physicians for professional consultation. Contact them at:

5600 S. Quebec, Ste. 109-A
Englewood, CO 80111
Phone: 303-779-4833, 303-770-2526
www.asbp.org

Federal Trade Commission offers a number of pamphlets on avoiding diet scams and ripoffs. Contact them at:

Consumer Response Center
600 Pennsylvania Ave., NW
Washington, DC 20580
www.ftc.gov

The Gold Coast Cure
By Dr. Andrew Larson and Ivy Ingram Larson
Published by Health Communications Inc.

National Institute of Diabetes and Digestive and Kidney Diseases Weight-Control Information Network (WIN) offers publications, including fact sheets, brochures, article reprints, and conference and workshop proceedings. They also offer a program called *Sisters Together: Move More, Eat Better,* which encourages Black women to maintain their weight by increasing their physical activity and eating healthy foods. Contact WIN at:

877-946-4627
www.niddk.nih.gov/health/nutrit/win.htm

National Weight Control Registry has identified more than four thousand individuals who have lost significant amounts of weight and kept it off for long periods of time. Their Web site offers success stories and other resources for weight loss. Contact them at:

800-606-NWCR (800-606-6927)
www.nwcr.ws

Obesity Education Initiative provides information on assessing your risk for developing weight-related diseases, as well as advice on losing weight. Contact them at:

National Heart, Lung, and Blood Institute
301-592-8573
http://rover.nhlbi.nih.gov/health/public/heart/obesity/ lose_wt/

Shape Up America! offers a "10,000 Steps" walking program, as well as information on childhood obesity and other weight-related topics. Visit their Web site at:

www.shapeup.org

The Surgeon General's Call to Action to Prevent and Decrease Overweight and Obesity is a report that outlines strategies that communities can use in helping to address the problems. The report is available at: *www.surgeongeneral.gov/topics/obesity/*

Who is Jack Canfield,
Co-creator of *Chicken Soup for the Soul*®?

Jack Canfield is one of America's leading experts in the development of human potential and personal effectiveness. He is both a dynamic, entertaining speaker and a highly sought-after trainer. Jack has a wonderful ability to inform and inspire audiences toward increased levels of self-esteem and peak performance. He has authored or coauthored numerous books, including *Dare to Win, The Aladdin Factor, 100 Ways to Build Self-Concept in the Classroom, Heart at Work* and *The Power of Focus*. His latest book is *The Success Principles*.

www.jackcanfield.com

Who is Mark Victor Hansen,
Co-creator of *Chicken Soup for the Soul*®?

In the area of human potential, no one is more respected than Mark Victor Hansen. For more than thirty years, Mark has focused solely on helping people from all walks of life reshape their personal vision of what's possible. His powerful messages of possibility, opportunity and action have created powerful change in thousands of organizations and millions of individuals worldwide. He is a prolific writer of bestselling books such as *The One Minute Millionaire, The Power of Focus, The Aladdin Factor* and *Dare To Win*.

www.markvictorhansen.com

Who is Andrew Larson, M.D.?

Andrew Larson, M.D., is a general surgeon practicing in Palm Beach County, Florida. He has special interests in preventive health care, nutrition, endocrine surgery, laparoscopic surgery and bariatric (obesity) surgery. Dr. Larson earned his medical degree from the University of Pennsylvania and has trained at some of the nation's most prestigious institutions, including New York's Memorial Sloan-Kettering Cancer Center. His research has been published in internationally distributed medical journals and presented at conferences sponsored by nationally prominent medical societies. He is affiliated with the American Medical Association, the American Society for Bariatric Surgery, the Society of Laparoendoscopic Surgeons, the Society of American Gastrointestinal Endoscopic Surgeons, the International Federation for the Surgery of Obesity, and the American College of Surgeons. He and his wife, Ivy Ingram Larson, are the coauthors of *The Gold Coast Cure,* published by Health Communications Inc.

Who is Celia Slom Vimont (writer)?

Celia Slom Vimont is a health and medical writer. A graduate of the Columbia School of Journalism, she has written for magazines, newspapers and wire services for both consumers and physicians. The former Director of Editorial Services for the American Lung Association, Celia served as in-house editor for books on asthma and smoking cessation for the association, and continues to write about a variety of lung health issues. Celia lives in New York City with her husband and son.

More Chicken Soup

Many of the stories in this book were submitted by readers just like you. If you would like more information on submitting a story, visit our Web site at *www. chickensoup.com.* If you do not have Web access, we can also be reached at:

Chicken Soup for the Soul
P.O. Box 30880, Santa Barbara, CA 93130
Fax: 805-563-2945

Contributors

John Bardinelli is a freelance writer and author currently working out of Iowa. More information on his work may be found on his Web site at *http://www.bardinelli.com.*

Harriet Cooper is a freelance humorist and essayist living in Toronto, Canada. Her humor, essays, articles, short stories and poetry have appeared in newspapers, magazines, Web sites, newsletters, anthologies, radio and a coffee can. She specializes in writing about family, relationships, cats, psychology and health. She can be reached at: *harcoop@hotmail.com.*

Suzan Davis found that the weight of mankind's future was not only upon her shoulders, but much of it had spread over her body. She wasn't going to take it lying down on the couch and founded an inline skating club called *Babes on Blades,* primarily for women over forty. *Babes on Blades: Drop Physical, Mental and Spiritual Flab Thru Inline Skating* skidded into the public in 2002, depicting models from 29 to 60, in sizes S, M and XXL—just like her readers. Suzan is also contributor to half a dozen anthologies including *Chicken Soup for the Inspired Women's Soul.* Suzan's public relations company promotes exercise and healthy living around the country. She lives in Granite Bay, California, with two charming children and two naughty, bad dogs. Suzan swears life begins after forty. Contact her at *suzandavis@surewest.net.*

Marilyn Eudaly, originally from Missouri, now lives in Texas with her husband and faithful dog Hairy Truman. Her daughter, who is mentioned here, lives nearby and is her writing mentor. Marilyn is a member of Romance Writers of America and just starting her writing career.

Jacquelyn B. Fletcher is a full-time freelance writer who has written hundreds of magazine articles in addition to nonfiction books, young adult fiction, brochures, Web content and a variety of other projects in the name of her motto: Will Write for Food. Contact her at *jacquebfletcher@aol.com.*

Jim Hammill is a business analyst with ANALYTIC*i* in New York. He lives in Caldwell, New Jersey, with wife Astrida and has two sons,

Chris and Greg. Jim loves singing bass with the locally popular a capella group Wide Variety. You can email Jim from the group's Web site, *http://www.widevariety.com.*

Georgia A. Hubley retired after 20 years in financial management to write her memoirs. She's a frequent contributor to the *Chicken Soup for the Soul* series and numerous national magazines and newspapers. She has two grown sons and resides with her husband in Henderson, Nevada. Contact her at *GEOHUB@aol.com.*

Vicki Jeffries is a homemaker and mother of four young children: Nathaniel, Alexander, Amanda, and Christian.

Mary Mooney, while living in Jakarta, Indonesia, for three years, conducted Team Building workshops throughout Asia, was a professional advisor to the public relations departments of several five-star hotels and the editor of the American Women's Association of Indonesia magazine. A certified multicultural diversity trainer, an actress (averaging one film a month) and a playwright, her piece "Memento" was published in *Chicken Soup for the Soul of America* following the 9/11 tragedy. Please contact her at *mooneym@erols.com* or *fredamooney@hotmail.com.*

Kirstein Mortensen, a public relations professional and writer from Rochester, New York, is the co-author of *Outwitting Dogs* (Lyons Press, Dec. 2004), a book on using rewards-based techniques for dog training, and the author of an upcoming novel. She welcomes e-mails at *MortensenKirsten@aol.com.*

Mary Silver lives in Montreal, Canada. Now that she is no longer concentrating on dieting, she has more time and energy to spend with her friends and family. She enjoys walking, reading and playing with her cat, Puss Puss. This is her first published story. She can be reached at: *marcoop27@hotmail.com.*

Joyce Stark lives in North East Scotland and works for the Community Mental Health. Her hobby is writing about people around her and those she meets on her travels in the USA. She is currently working on a series to introduce very young children to a second language. E-mail: *joric.stark@virgin.net.*

Ken Swarner is author of *Whose Kids Are These Anyway?* (Penguin/ Putnam). He can be seen at *www.kenswarner.com.*

Amy Westlake, N.D., a board-certified naturopathic physician, earned her medical degree from Bastyr University in Seattle, Washington. Dr. Westlake resides in Huntsville, Alabama, with her husband, Rodney, and their daughter, Lucy.

Lydia Witherspoon is a writer based in South Florida. When she's not busy working, she loves long walks and lounging at the beach.